Dry Eye Disease Treatment in the Year 2020

Rolando Toyos, MD

Dry Eye Disease Treatment in the Year 2020

Edited
By
Barbie "Dr. Jay" Jodoin, OD

Contributions
By
Melissa Morrison Toyos, MD
Barbie Jodoin, OD

Disclosure

I or the contributors to this book have had research support or have completed consulting for several companies whose products may or may not be mentioned in this book. We are including a list of all companies past or present for which we have had any financial contract for full disclosure.

American Society of Cataract and Refractive Surgery

Joint Commission on Allied Health Personnel

Quantum Ocular Bioscience

Dermamed

Lumenis

Arteriocyte

Alcon

Novartis

Bausch and Lomb

Valeant

Allergan

Pharmacia

Oculus

Young

TearLab

Shire

Pfizer

Merck

Abbott

Santen

To my loving family that inspire me:

Melissa Morrison Toyos, Eva Hammock-Toyos, Allison Cable, Catherine Cable, Lt. Col Ruben George Toyos, Binnie Toyos

Acknowledgements

My Mentors Past and Present

Francisco "Papi" Batista, Coach Pat Ryan, Dr. William Wallace, Roger Parkin, Professor Howard Bern, Professor Lee Shulman

All those people in the Dry Eye Disease trenches with me

Dr. Melissa Morrison Toyos, Dr. Haylie Mulliniks, Nikki Barbee, Dr. Dustin Briscoe, Dr. Jessica Armstrong, Dr. Barbie Jodoin, Dr. Marcie Daniels, Dr. Jenny Duncan, Dr. Kristal Jones, Cheryl Cox, Roger Parkin, Durenda Camp, Itay Mayer, Mark Pinsley, Ginger Pruden Hodulik, Dr. William McGill, Janice Prestwood, Pat Mathey, my incredible staff past and present, and all the patients that believed in our clinic.

Table of Contents

Foreword

Introduction

Chapter 1: Dry Eye Disease

Chapter 2: Intense Pulse Light

Chapter 3: The Q

Chapter 4: Diet & Supplements

Chapter 5: Drop therapy: Non-medicated and Medicated

Chapter 6: Pain

Chapter 7: Surgery

Chapter 8:Skin

Chapter 9: Aging

Chapter 10: Environment

Chapter 11: Treatments that didn't make the cut

Chapter 12: The Future in Dry Eye

Bibliography

Foreword

When Dr. Toyos suggested that I write the foreword to his book on Dry Eye Treatment, I was both pleased and honored. Pleased because, as a Dry Eye disease patient, I understand the discomfort, daily distraction and even pain that can ensue from this disease. After receiving Dr. Toyos,' IPL treatment, I found immediate relief. I was honored because, as owner of a biotechnology company invested in the Intense Pulse Light (IPL) platform, I have worked with Dr. Toyos to help improve IPL technology for use in his groundbreaking treatments.

While most physicians involved with ocular medicine now accept IPL treatment as a gold standard for helping to resolve the symptoms of Dry Eye disease, this was not always the case. After my treatment with Dr. Toyos in 2007, we worked to formulate a plan to educate other physicians about this trail-blazing treatment. I observed his dedicated research methods, developing innovative protocols and treating patients. Because he is an advocate for the best care for his patients, I saw people around the world reaching out to him for treatment. I also witnessed the perseverance he demonstrated in enlightening the medical field about this revolutionary treatment.

As a friend, I have encouraged Dr. Toyos to share his information with countless other Dry Eye sufferers. Many individuals who are plagued with the symptoms of Dry Eye disease may not even realize their undiagnosed condition, nor understand the ease of treatment that can change the quality of their lives. This book contains groundbreaking research and practical information that is essential reading for Dry Eye disease sufferers.

Roger Parkin, CEO

Vision Medical, Inc.

"Time makes more converts than reason. It is error only, and not truth, that shrinks from inquiry."

      Thomas Paine (1737- 1809)

Introduction

      Medical textbooks can be complicated in a time where information is at your fingertips. Medical discoveries you plan to place in a book now could be disproven, blasé, or worse, outdated by the time the book is printed. So, even though I have started this book on Dry Eye Disease (DED) many times before, I never felt that it would be more useful than a blog, video, or tweet. I have been in the center of a paradigm shift in the treatment of Dry Eye Disease with my discovery of Intense Pulse Light (IPL) and other light treatments as a solution to the problem. When I began writing a book on the treatment, I stopped and opted for a video instead because I thought it would get the information out to the general public quicker. My thinking was by the time a book would come out so many physicians would be utilizing IPL that the information would be ubiquitous. Well, I was completely wrong. My video is close to 10 years old, and it has only been now that IPL has been in the conversation as a treatment modality in research journals.

      New ideas in medicine are not like new ideas in the social media world where a woman stating, "Nobody got time for that", can go viral in a day. A paradigm shift in medicine takes years to develop and implement. Even in the face of inarguable evidence, the scientific skeptics will be out in full force to discredit research. The United States Food and Drug Administration, FDA, states that it takes on average 12 years and $350 million to bring a drug from the laboratory to the pharmacy shelf. Even once a drug is approved, it still will take time for the medical community to adopt. We can chalk this up to the fact that, as scientists, we are taught to question everything, but I am afraid that it has become more complicated than a healthy mistrust of information. Science has been corrupted by money. Now, impartial researchers and clinicians are paid vast sums of money by various corporations and agencies to prove a self-serving agenda correct instead of applying the Socratic method to a problem. Is it surprising? Labs, studies, and the ability to bring a new drug or technology to market can be expensive. Researchers are under pressure to generate enough revenue to make their employment relevant.   If a company can make a billion dollars a year on a medication, is it a big stretch to think that they are going to employ scientists and clinicians to advance their enterprise?

In the environment of pseudo-science, I learned the hard way that a good idea can take years to filter out to the patients that need it. I was naïve to think that a book I would write today would be obsolete by the time it hit the presses. I researched IPL for 8 years after initially making the discovery before I presented a technology and treatment protocol to other physicians. There is pseudo-science being practiced by physicians, so I can't lay all the blame on corporations, universities, and government agencies. In dry eye disease community, I have seen where a doctor will promote an idea to the world like it is fact. For example, I am very weary of a doctor that presents a medication or technology as a cure for dry eye disease.   Why am I skeptical? Because I have been burned several times listening to a physician's hyperbole only to find out later that they had a huge financial stake in the product that they were hawking to other physicians and the public. In today's world, your words and writings will follow you for a long time. If a doctor is untruthful, his ideas will follow him, but the patients will not. I often say that I do not receive dirty looks from my colleagues because I have been able to keep my integrity by never selling out. In turn, there are a group of clinicians and scientists that I follow as well because they have proven their integrity. I compare the pretenders to Icarus – they rise very quickly on hot air and reach the light of truth, finally burning and crashing to the ground with the reality that their idea didn't match their bravado.

I have written this book to give dry eye sufferers understanding and hope. As a former teacher, my goal is to simply explain how I handle dry eye disease. I spend time going around the country training doctors in Dry Eye Disease and attending research meetings. I have the privilege of hearing the latest and the future treatments that are available. I also attend scientific meetings that are not geared to eye disease but may spark an idea that can translate into an eye treatment. It was this open mindedness that led me to bring Intense Pulse Light to Ophthalmology but do not think that we have stood still with this invention. We understand that innovation advances lead to better ways to treat a multifactorial disease like Dry Eye. I hope to arm you with information that you can use to achieve relief now and in the future.

Before you begin my book, I ask that you listen to an old story that I adapted for our purposes. There was a patient who was very successful, smart, had accumulated great wealth, but was suffering from Dry Eye Disease. He was able to travel the world to visit every DED specialist around. He learned many things from talking to these doctors and researching his disease on the worldwide web. He could not find relief and wanted to see this one specific DED specialist that many thought was wise. The specialist had trained many and helped many patients from far and near, never turning someone who wanted to learn away. When he arrived at the clinic for his exam, he began to show off in front of the staff about all the DED knowledge he had accumulated. He even began to scold the staff members about the way they were performing the exams. The specialist heard this and invited the man to come have tea with him in the kitchen.

"Why have you come to see me today?" asked the specialist.

"I have come today to ask you to teach me about DED. Open my mind and enlighten me," said the patient.

The doctor smiled and began to pour the tea in his cup. He poured and poured, overfilling the cup. The tea overflowed beyond the rim of the cup and on to the patient's clothes. Finally, the visitor yelled, "Enough. You are spilling tea all over. Can't you see the cup is full?"

The specialist stopped pouring and smiled at his guest. "You are like this tea cup, so full that nothing more can be added. Come back to me when the cup is empty."

Empty your mind and begin to read, <u>Dry Eye Disease Treatment in the Year 2020</u>.

"The cure of many diseases is unknown to the physicians of Hellas, because they are ignorant of the whole, which ought to be studied also; for the part can never be well unless the whole is well …. This is the great error of our day in the treatment of the human body, that the physicians separate the soul from the body."

Plato (427-347 B.C.)

Chapter 1: Dry Eye Disease

It is as true today as it was then. I added Plato's quote to my first book in 1994 for prospective medical students because I believed then what I know now that you have to adopt a holistic approach to patient care. Too often into today's health care environment, a doctor would like to give a patient a prescription for a medicine and tell them to go on their way without discussing the environment and the health choices that they are making every minute that affects their disease. DED is no different. If we understand the underlying pathophysiological problems of DED, then you can make better lifestyle choices to improve your situation.

Dry eye disease is an inflammatory disease that involves skin, glands, nervous system, and eyes (Figure 1). I put the eyes last in that statement because most medical professionals focus on the eyes when dealing with patients with DED complaints and forget the rest. I teach that DED is a skin and gland problem that affects the eyes. For a healthy functioning eye, you need a normal tear film.

Figure 1. The eye. (Shutter Stock)

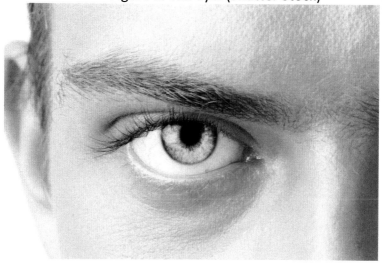

A tear consists of three parts (Figure 2): 1. A mucous layer (protein) that coats the eye and is produced by goblet cells on the conjunctiva. 2. An aqueous layer (water) that is produced by the lacrimal gland and provides water, electrolytes, antibodies, lipocalin, lactoferrin, lysozyme, and lacritin. 3. A lipid layer (fat) that is produced by the meibomian glands on the lid margin. All three parts are necessary to have a normal tear. The easiest way to think of the three components is as individual layers stacked on top of one another. The mucous layer sits on the cornea with the water layer making the bulk of the tear in the center and the fat layer on the outside. The cornea, unlike many parts of our body, normally does not have blood vessels in it enabling us to have a clear window to the world. For the cornea to survive, we rely on nutrients from our tears to supply the important factors that a body part needs to survive. The nutrients come from the aqueous layer. The tear needs to stay on the eye long enough to provide those nutrients. The fatty layer keeps the tear from evaporating too quickly. The tear also plays an important role in vision.

Figure 2. Tear Film (Can Stock Photo)

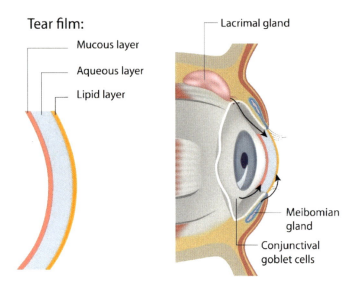

I often explain the tear and vision using my windshield wiper analogy. If you were driving in your car on a dry sunny day and you had the windshield wipers going without any rain, then eventually those wipers would cause scratches on the windshield and decrease visibility. On a rainy day, every time the wiper goes across you have a nice clear view as the water is spread evenly across the windshield. We are constantly producing tears, and each time we blink, it affords us a great view as the tear is spread evenly on the cornea. However just like the wiper on a dry day, if you do not produce a perfectly balanced tear, then each time you blink, you could create micro scratches and dry spots on the cornea that will decrease vision.

We have pain sensory nerves on the cornea that are activated when these dry spots become worse. These nerves are connected to the pupillary reflex. This is the reason patients who have injury to the cornea from DED often are light sensitive because when the pupil constricts or dilates, the cornea nerves are activated, causing pain. When we have a patient with a cornea injury, we dilate the pupil, essentially freezing the pupil so that the pain is minimized with immobility of the iris.

If any of the glands are dysfunctional, then it could lead to DED and pain. Goblet cells can be affected by injury to the conjunctiva. A common injury to the conjunctiva is due to access exposure to the elements, like sun and wind. We often see scarring in the conjunctiva, called pingecula, with longstanding exposure and dry eye. When the scarring begins to invade the cornea, we call that a ptyergium. Unless there is an acute injury from chemicals, we rarely see DED caused just by Goblet cell deterioration. The longstanding inflammation of DED can begin to cause a decrease in goblet cells. Certain medications and artificial tears have been shown to increase goblet cell density, but I have yet to see one of these medications affect DED symptoms.

Some autoimmune diseases can cause lacrimal gland dysfunction, hampering the basal tear formation. I tend to think of the lacrimal gland like a sponge soaking wet with water. When the eye is too dry, the only defense that your body has is to squeeze all the water from the sponge on to the eye. This is the reason why many dry eye patients complain of watery eyes. The only thing the lacrimal gland can provide in a dry eye situation is saline tears without any nutrients. These are called reflex tears and are produced when the eye is exposed to irritants, like pepper spray. A tear with an abnormally high percentage of water only helps to wash irritants away and protects in a short-term emergency response but does not help vision or the health of the cornea. The lacrimal gland also produces the emotional watery tear. Some studies show that crying tears contain special hormones, triggering emotional feelings. Sjogren's Disease is the most common autoimmune disease that can cause decrease in aqueous production.

By far, the most common type of DED is meibomian gland dysfunction. The Meibomian Gland (MG) produces an olive oil-like secretion called meibum. The lipids are a combination of wax esters, cholesteryl esters, fatty acids, and proteins. The MG produces a unique long-chain fatty acid that is insoluble in water. Without the correct composition of meibum, the tear evaporates quicker than normal. The time it takes for a tear to evaporate is called the tear break up time, TBUT. In the past, it has been measured by doctor observation, but recently, automated technology has been used. In our clinic, we measured TBUT in normal young people to be anywhere from 10 seconds up to 30 seconds. Less than 10 seconds is considered abnormal, meaning a sign that the gland is producing an irregular lipid. Once an abnormal fatty layer is produced, not only is the tear film disrupted, the health of the cornea is compromised. Currently, researchers are studying the composition of meibum in normal and disease states to determine the difference in a science called lipidomics.

When measuring the tear film as a whole in disease states, we have discovered that there can be a whole host of inflammatory mediators. For the past several years at the International Society of Ophthalmic and Therapeutics (ISOPT) annual meeting, we have presented several of these inflammatory byproducts. When reading articles on inflammatory biomarkers in tears, you will hear names like interleukins (IL 1 through 9), matrix metalloproteinases (MMP 9), cytokines, T cells, tissue necrosis factor TNF, iCAM, to name a few. Do not get bogged down with the alphabet soup of inflammation because as we speak, more inflammatory mediators are found every day. All of these inflammatory cells lead to the same result – dry, irritated, red, swollen, painful eyes and lids.

The inflammation leads to more dysfunction of the glands and cells that make up the tear film, leading to an increased risk of infection. Without the antimicrobial properties of our tear film, the normal bacteria and parasites that live on our skin can overgrow. In an environment of infection and inflammation, it is no wonder that dry eye disease progressively becomes worse over time if left untreated. As inflammation and infection overwhelm an anatomical structure, the nerves become more sensitized, increasing pain. Many DED patients describe pain on every blink as the lid moves across the cornea. Many patients have discussed their pain with their healthcare professionals without much attention being paid to their suffering because it was seen as a nuisance disease, but with the disease cycle in mind, you can understand why DED patients suffer. Other body parts with the same pathology received more attention and focus. For example, chronic knee inflammation brought on several medications, treatments, and surgeries. When I began specializing in Dry Eye Disease in 1998, there was not even a medication for the problem.

The complexity of DED as opposed to other inflammatory processes is that it is in the area of the body that serves a complex sense and has many parts that have to work correctly to give a desired result. Just think that the tear is created by three different structures all to support a special part of the body – the cornea. The cornea is a clear structure that does not have blood vessels to provide nutrition but relies on the tear and the aqueous humor (fluid produced in the eye). The outer layer of the cornea (epithelium) like skin is constantly regenerating. The epithelium of the cornea has more nerve endings per capita than any other structure in the body. The cornea is considered an immune privileged site because of the lack of vessels, which is why it has such a high success rate with transplantation.

With tear glands located within the skin, underneath the skin, and on the eye itself, it is easy to see why many factors affect the tear film. It is not a stretch to think that our environment, diet, genetics, medication use, hygiene, occupation, age, hormones, and sex all play a role in our tear production and the severity of Dry Eye Disease. A holistic approach to the problem is the only way to attack this multifactorial problem. If your eye doctor didn't spend a good amount of time listening and probing into your medical, social, family history before the physical exam, then she missed the opportunity to really solve your DED dilemma. If in physical exam, the doctor looked at your eye for a diagnosis without taking into account your skin and glands, he missed one of the more important parts of the diagnosis. I had a professor tell me early in my career the only way to find out what is wrong with the patient is to talk to the patient. He was pointing this out in the beginning of the use of the MRI. He saw too many doctors eschewing the traditional ways of medicine like obtaining patient history and physical exam, instead relying on technology to make the diagnosis. Technology in healthcare is to aid the clinician, not take the place of the clinician. This is an important point in the DED space because many doctors are adopting tests like biomarkers to make the diagnosis of dry eye. These tests can be expensive for the patient and our healthcare system. Recently, I read an article published in a throw away magazine where a doctor discussed the several expensive tests that she made a patient perform before diagnosing dry eye, when the patient experienced all the classic symptoms of dry eye as well as physical signs of dry eye. The tests she ran were inconclusive at best. She decided to treat the patient. In reality, the patient was going to be treated for dry eye based on history and physical exam. Did the patient really have to pay for all those tests?

As I mentioned before, more tests are coming to the market every day for Dry Eye Disease. There is a biomarker that measures the inflammatory mediator, MMP 9. There is another test that measures tear osmolarity because, in theory, patients with dry eye will have a higher tear osmolarity than a determined normal. The problem with both these tests and any future tests is that they are not specific for DED. As my wife, Dr. Melissa Toyos, likes to say there isn't a simple yes or no pregnancy test in dry eye. With the complexity of the system that I have described, do we really believe that we will find such a test? Every year, we find new biomarkers that are elevated in Dry Eye. Will one of these be the specific one that is elevated a certain amount in DED that we can use as a screening test? Will we find that a certain amount of genetic markers that will tell us about each of the different glands that make up the tear will be revealed? Is there a marker for the lacrimal gland, another for the meibomian gland, and yet another for the goblet cell?

In this book, I am more concerned in treatment and not diagnosis because I have written this book for you, the DED patient. You know you have DED, and that is why you are reading this now. You want relief, and you want to know all the ways you can get it now and in the future. You will not find a magic bullet here. I will not tell you that you will take a pill or drop, and this will all go away. What I can tell you is that patients in our Dry Eye clinic have found relief when other clinics have failed. When something is not working for them, we have other treatments that may work better. I tell patients that I have never found one artificial tear that all patients agree on, but each patient has found a tear that they use to make them feel better. Why is that? I believe it has to do with the pH, composition, active and inactive ingredients, and how this all interacts with the current natural tear that the patient is producing. The more important idea is that one size does not fit all when it comes to DED treatment. Since we are dealing with so many different mechanisms, it may be that one treatment modality may not be enough.

So read every treatment I discuss in this book and adopt the ones that you want to or can. If a treatment is not available yet, I will make that distinction in the discussion. I will also be talking about treatments that are way in the future. The reason I named it Dry Eye Disease Treatment in the year 2020 was to reflect some of the treatments in the future. The current census states that the average man will live to 82, and the average woman will live to 86. So you can look forward to a future where treatments will improve and more relief is on the way. Do not despair, we have concrete treatments for you now and evolved ones for the future.

"We can easily forgive a child who is afraid of the dark; the real tragedy of life is when men are afraid of the light."

Plato (427-347 B.C.)

Chapter 2: Intense Pulse Light

I am starting with the Intense Pulse Light treatment for DED because it is the procedure and technology that I invented and perfected. It has taught me the most on the struggles that a researcher faces bringing a paradigm shift to the world of medicine. I recently lectured at my alma mater, Stanford University, to the student Optical Society of America, OSA. In attendance were biomedical researchers, physicians, undergraduate and graduate students who attended the meeting to hear how their innovations could be translated into medical discovery. They also wanted to understand the struggles faced on the road to invention.

Archimedes stepped into in a bathtub one day and realized that the water level rose, helping him understand that the volume of water displaced must equal to the volume of the part of his body he submerged. When he realized his discovery, he yelled, "Eureka", and jumped out of the tub and ran naked through the streets of Syracuse. My "Eureka" moment happened in my clinic during work hours, so there was no running naked through the streets of Tennessee.

In 2001, my clinic was beginning to grow, and I had an opportunity to purchase an old pediatric clinic that was divided into several pods. We decided that we were going to place an Aesthetics clinic in one of our pods. During that time, many new innovations were being brought to market that allowed patients to improve their appearance without having to undergo traditional surgery. At the time, I was already performing lid surgeries, including blepharoplasty and lid lifts. I love technology, and I was excited to expand into new areas of Ophthalmology. Many of my Lasik patients were also asking for treatments such as Botox and facial rejuvenation technology. We invested in many technologies, such as Erbium and YAG lasers as well as Intense Pulse Light (IPL). At the time, it was known that IPL could help remove the redness from skin in rosacea patients.

I would send rosacea patients over to the aesthetics side, where our nurse would treat the face with IPL. I would see these patients back in our clinic and ask how the treatments were going. Some of the patients stated that since they started treatment with IPL, their dry eye symptoms had improved. The tear film in these patients improved, and their lid margins and meibomian glands looked better. More importantly, I could see that the meibum secretions had a more normal consistency. Eureka!!!!

I was a James Scholar in medical school from 1990 to 1994, and my research in trauma surgery concentrated on the role of non-steroidal anti-inflammatory drugs to help patients survive post-operative repair of trauma. I learned that inflammation causes dysfunction in several organs in the body, including the eye. As a resident in Ophthalmology at Northwestern University, I continued my work studying inflammation, this time focusing on the eye. I began to attend and present research at the Association for Research in Vision and Ophthalmology annual meeting. You could find some poster boards on inflammation, but the most interesting were research papers on how cyclosporine therapy (an immunosuppressant drug used in rheumatoid arthritis and to prevent transplant rejection) helped control inflammation of the eye and lacrimal gland in human and animal models. These studies that I was following at ARVO from 1995 to 1998 on cyclosporine began addressing the role of inflammation in disease. At that time, DED was called dry eye syndrome, and no one was addressing it. Even the studies on cyclosporine would usually have conjunctivitis in their title, not Dry Eye. The definition of Dry Eye by the National Eye Institute stated "Dry Eye is a disorder of the tear film due to tear deficiency or excessive evaporation which causes damage to the interpalpebral ocular surface and is associated with symptoms of ocular discomfort.[1]" There was no mention of inflammation in the definition of Dry Eye. Eventually, a few dry eye experts like myself understood that dry eye was an inflammatory disease and began to treat it with anti-inflammatory drops, including cyclosporine topical drops prepared by a compound pharmacy. In 1999, cyclosporine drops under the name Restasis was first rejected by the FDA, finally winning approval in 2002.

Even though inflammation was not part of the official definition, I knew that to relieve dry eye disease you would have to control inflammation. If some of my DED patients were improving with IPL, then that meant that IPL was controlling inflammation. I have been conducting research since my college days at Berkeley and Stanford back in the late 80's and what I learned very quickly is that you will have many Eureka moments; some work out, and some do not. If you think the idea is impactful enough, you have to scrutinize it with research. After seeing a few patients with improvement after IPL, I decided to devote my time to research the connection. As stated before, very few doctors were devoting their time to dry eye disease; even the early researchers of Restasis were actually looking for a drop to control allergies. Most doctors saw this as a nuisance disease that didn't warrant time or research money, but I was seeing something different in our clinic. The dry eye patients were the most miserable about their situation. It reminded me of the back pain clinic that I staffed when I did my orthopedics rotation in medical school. I thought I may just have the answer here.

I began to treat dry eye patients myself for free with IPL. I experimented with energy levels and pulses on different skin types, including my own. We learned very quickly that the use of IPL would not be a general treatment that parameters and protocols did not matter in the effectiveness of treatment. Intense Pulse Light (figure 3) is a Xenon flash lamp that generates a broad wavelength of light. You can apply cut off filters, usually sapphire glass, that will block certain wavelengths of light and allow higher wavelengths of light to pass on to the skin. You can pulse that light, varying the on and off pulses in milliseconds. The lighter the skin the more energy and fewer pulses you can utilize. The darker the skin the less energy and the more pulses are administered. The wavelength of visible light allowed to pass is around 550nanometers and higher. This wavelength is absorbed by skin, blood cells, glands, and pigment. The more pigment or blood vessels you have, the more energy will be absorbed. Our first group of DED patients treated were rosacea patients because the fine abnormal blood vessels (telangiectasias) on the outer layer of their skin absorb IPL and generate heat, which coagulates these vessels. We hypothesized that IPL was working on these patients because it was closing of abnormal blood vessels that secrete inflammatory mediators that hamper the normal function of the meibomian gland, but what we found early on was that some patients that didn't have rosacea but had MGD also were helped with IPL. As I treated a more diverse group of patients with varying protocols and parameters, I began to see more consistent improvement. We may have something here.

Figure 3. IPL treatment (Toyos Clinic)

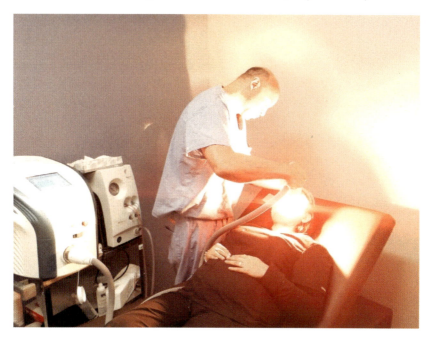

We completed a thorough case report that we submitted to the different journals. I learned very quickly that introducing technology that most Ophthalmologists have never heard of was going to be difficult for them to accept. Our first case study in 2002 was not accepted by any publications. We kept researching, improving the treatment, and refining the parameters. I gave my first concept lecture on dry eye disease and IPL in 2002 before the Restasis approval to a room full of eye doctors. No one understood the lecture. Then, in 2003, Restasis gained approval, and a few dry eye talks began to spring up at our national meetings. The role of inflammation began to be talked about in connection with DED. We finally had one of our case studies accepted in 2003 for publication. The American Society of Cataract and Refractive Surgery committed to publishing a case study. They also honored us with a research grant to study IPL as a dry eye treatment. We presented a prospective study on IPL for DED in 2005. In that study, we showed positive results but not clinically significant results. Our protocol and technology was not perfected.

Research requires time, dedication, and funding. I had our research department turn down other projects so that we could concentrate on IPL for dry eye. Before my first major presentation, I went to all of the Intense Pulse Light manufacturers to discuss our idea. Most companies were not interested in the idea because they did not see a big need of a treatment for dry eye. Some companies didn't feel like eye doctors would utilize IPL. Others didn't have understanding of the connection between their technology and the eye. A few companies allowed me to utilize their technology for a brief time, but it was a temporary loan to see if I would buy their IPL system. I purchased a few and kept researching. As I have stated many times, we decided not to charge patients until I felt we had a perfected treatment. This is important because now many IPL companies are jumping into dry eye making claims that their technology can duplicate our treatment. The problem is that not all IPL systems are the same. Also, you have to do thorough research to find the right parameters and protocol for each skin type. Our big break came in 2006 when a manufacturer listened to my modifications and parameters. Also, a few companies invested in advancing the technology. One of the major problems with simple IPL systems is that after each treatment, the power (fluence) produced by the Xenon flash lamp would degrade so you would have less power, meaning that a setting you used at one time would not give you the same effect the next time. You would constantly have to increase your settings to achieve the same result.

I worked with the new company for 2 years before we had a finished product with proven results. Again, we completed several prospective and retrospective studies showing improvement in the tear film, lids, skin, glands, and TBUT. We submitted our studies to various journals who rejected our research. Most editors stated that they didn't understand how IPL could possibly work to help DED. During that time, I was able to present the results at several international meetings. The advantage of a lecture, as opposed to a paper, is that you can explain the treatment and answer questions. The ability to answer questions for someone with no experience in light treatments is important because you can explain the science until the "light bulb" turns on in their head.

Why does Intense Pulse Light (figure 4) treat DED? In 2001, many of the scientific research that had been done with light for the human body was not available for the general public and even the scientific community. Most people have not heard of non-profit organizations that have been studying light for decades, like the Society of Photo-Optical Instrumentation Engineers (SPIE)[2], an international society advancing an interdisciplinary approach to the science and application of light, or the Optical Society of America (OSA)[3] that advances the study of light – optics and photonics – in theory and application, by means of publishing, organizing conferences and exhibitions, and partnering with industry on education. The study of light has been ongoing, including for the use in medicine. Many of the studies have been conducted by NASA[4] and were classified at the time. A novel written by Carl Sagan in the 80's called Contact, which was developed into a movie with Jodie Foster in the 90's, showed that NASA had been studying the effects of space on the human body and have been researching how to counteract its effects. In the movie, one of the characters contracts cancer and is given a short time to live. The character is a billionaire, and to prolong his life, he pays the Russians to let him live on the space station because in space, cells slow down, including the growth of his cancer cells. The character lives in the space station well past the time that he was given on earth. In reality, NASA discovered that in space, the mitochondria (the powerhouse of the cell) and other cellular processes slow down, which would cause health problems including aging of the skin. Because of this, they began experimenting with certain wavelengths of light to counter act this phenomenon. The ability of light to stimulate the cellular processes, like mitochondria, to work better is called Photomodulation (some call it photobiomodulation). We witness photomodualtion when IPL stimulates the fibroblasts to produce collagen, making the skin look youthful and improved.

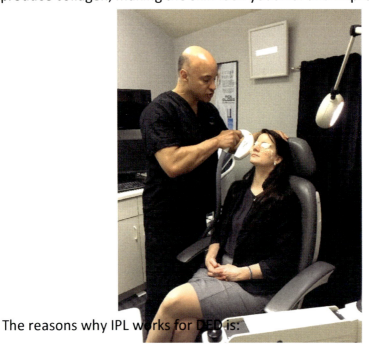

The reasons why IPL works for DED is:

1. The specific wavelength of light at the right parameters and protocol stimulates the cells of the Meibomian Gland to function normally. Many DED patients that have been

treated in our clinic possessing glands that have dropped out as seen by meibography[5] (technology that can take a picture of a gland that can show if it is functioning or not) have had rejuvenation with IPL treatments, restoring function. I no longer subscribe to the idea of scarred down glands. I prefer to say that the glands are dormant. We utilize IPL to photomodulate the cells of the Meibomian Gland leading to better meibum production.

2. IPL allows us to express glands of all of its abnormal contents. The particular wavelength of light used in IPL for DED has the ability to penetrate the inner layers of the skin where the Meibomian Glands are located, generating enough heat to melt the solid secretions in the dysfunctional glands[6]. Eyelid temperature is normally about 33 degree C (91degrees Fahrenheit). Abnormal meibum has a higher melting temperature than 33 degrees. Some warm compresses can raise the temperature of the lids by 5 degrees to 38 degrees C, but I have found, in the most severe cases of MGD, that this is not enough to even soften the abnormal meibum. A treatment like Lipiflow heats the inner lids to about 42.5 C which does melt the secretions, allowing mechanical expression. After IPL, you can achieve skin temperatures as high as 62 C. The advantage of IPL is that it is heating the skin from the dermal layer to the epidermal layer, which is opposite of a warm compress. We have found no better treatment to open the glands and melt the abnormal meibum effectively, making manual expression easy. Patients symptomatically feel better after an expression because you have unclogged a blocked gland. Now, any meibum produced can be released into the tear film, but the improvement of symptoms of any heat and expression procedure is short lived unless you can produce normal meibum. We had several patients that are not candidates that undergo serial warmth with expressions. Patients with moderate MGD will state that symptomatic

relief will last 3 weeks. We incorporated MG expression into our IPL procedure to give immediate short term relief to patients so that they would continue treatment until the complete photomodulation of the glands could be achieved.

3. Certain wavelengths of light have the ability to kill[7] - photodynamic[8] toxicity by oxidative damage - bacteria and parasites[9] on the skin. Intense Pulse Light robots, called Xenex, are used to disinfect hospital surgical and non-surgical rooms. During the Ebola crisis, when a hospital in the Dallas area received Ebola patients, they utilized the Xenex robot to disinfect their entire facility. It has long been known that IPL is an effective treatment of acne because it can kill the bacteria. We know that bacteria and parasites that are normally on our lid margin will overgrow when MGD occurs. The bacteria in question are Staphylococcus Epidermis and Aureus, P. Acnes, and Corynebacterium; the parasite is Demodex. The overgrowth of these bacteria can lead to the inflammation and infection of the lid margins, Blepharitis. DED and Blepharitis play the chicken and egg game of ocular surface disease. The microbes can release lipases, which breakdown our normal fatty acids in the tear film, leading to increased inflammatory cytokine release. The inflammatory mediators cause the gland dysfunction, leading to more microbial overgrowth that leads to more inflammation. We have seen where IPL for MGD (Figure 5) and DED decreases the bacteria and demodex, relieving Blepharitis.

Figure 5. MGD (Toyos Clinic)

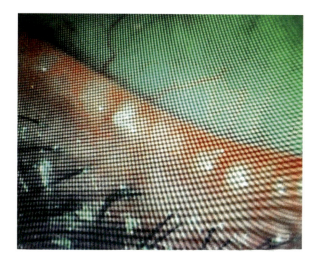

4. IPL was first used to close abnormal blood vessels (telangiectasias) in Rosacea. In MGD, we can see these telangiectasias on the lid margin. These blood vessels carry inflammatory cytokines to the area and the gland, causing poor functioning of the meibomian glands. Closing of telangiectasias at the lid margin improves the inflammation of the lids. Many patients tell me that they have seen other doctors, even Dermatologists, who have told them they do not have Rosacea. As Ophthalmologists, we have the ability to observe the thin skin around the lids and see these telangiectasias with our microscope called the Slit Lamp. These telangiectasias exist on the rest of the face, but they are not as easily seen since the skin of the rest of the face is thicker. We have the ability to diagnosis milder forms of Rosacea before other doctors with the slit lamp focused on the lids. As we age, our fibroblasts of our skin stop producing collagen, causing the epidermis to thin over time. Many patients will state they did not have rosacea when they were in their twenties, but in their thirties and beyond, they began to notice the changes. Nothing has changed except the thickness of the epidermis. They had rosacea before, but it was not diagnosed. I am more aggressive in diagnosing these milder forms of rosacea patients because I

know, left unchecked, that the disease will begin to disrupt the normal function of the Meibomian Glands. The light from IPL will be absorbed by the red blood cells, generating heat, and ultimately closing down of the abnormal blood vessels carrying the inflammatory mediators, decreasing the breakdown of the meibomian glands. If you can treat these patients at an earlier age, you can prevent some of damage that happens to the glands and eyes over time.

5. Some studies demonstrate that the skin can produce inflammatory mediators. One study showed that IPL reduces the amount of interleukin-9 that is produced on the skin. I have seen in acne patients have worsening of their dry eye and inflammation around the lids during outbreaks. When we apply IPL to their acne, not only does the skin condition subside, their dry eye signs and symptoms decrease. We have had a group of patients between the ages of 10 to 19 that have had severe acne rosacea skin disease (Figure 6), causing deleterious effects to the eye due to severe MGD. These patients exhibit ocular rosacea and abnormal vessels on the cornea so severe that the patients cannot keep their eyes open because of the pain of eye exposure. The patients have non-existent TBUT, preventing them from seeing. We have been able to treat these patients with IPL, calming the inflammation on the face and, more importantly, reversing the signs and symptoms of ocular rosacea. A 10 year old patient was brought in by her family 8 years ago at their wits end with bad acne and ocular rosacea. She had not opened her eyes in over 3 months because of the pain. Her cornea looked like a war zone with peripheral scarring, inflamed blood vessels invading the cornea, and a 1 second TBUT. After one IPL treatment, her condition improved, and she was able to open her eyes. Over the years, her corneas have developed normally, and the abnormal blood vessels have regressed. She returns periodically for IPL treatments, visiting more frequently

when she has an outbreak. We have many more patients like her in the same age group that have been controlled with IPL. The skin to gland to eye connection is strong and holds the key to treatment.

Figure 6. Acne Rosacea (Toyos Clinic)

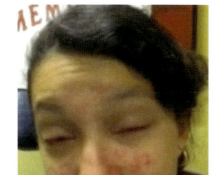

Several prestigious institutions and doctors have adopted my IPL treatment and technology into their practice and have experienced similar successful results to mine. Now, we have companies and doctors trying to utilize whatever non-descript IPL system that they can cheaply buy.   The problem with this approach is it ignores the eight years of research that our clinic conducted to bring the treatment to market in 2008. When IPL reached doctor's offices in 2000, the technology was basic in the sense that energy levels were not controlled, the pulses not easily programmable, and with increased use, the flash lamp would lose its power. It was used for facial rejuvenation and to close abnormal blood vessels in rosacea patients. How would a physician be able to tell what were the correct parameters to use on the face? We would have to perform a test spot on the skin by the ear, the tragus, and see if it turned a certain pinkish hue for you to determine that you had hit the right energy level, filter, and pulses for that machine. Once you determined the parameters, you could treat the rest of the face, but you could not treat around the lids because that thin skin would burn. Most doctors stayed away from the lids when treating. If the patient came for subsequent treatments, you would have to start over with a test spot because with increased use of the technology, the power would decrease in the bulb and your initial protocol for the patient would be too weak. You would constantly increase the programmed power on the IPL as time wore on. I remember in one patient I started with a fluence of 18 J/cm2, and after a year for the same treatment, I had to increase the power to 33 J/cm2 to achieve the same results because the lamp weakened. So we had to construct an IPL system that had a consistent energy.

Lumenis, the first company to bring IPL to the market, improved on their design and created the M22 IPL with Optimal Pulse Technology, ensuring that the fluence and power programmed match the output that the IPL generates. The technology self-calibrates to ensure correct powers every time. We now have the ability to customize the treatment for each individual knowing that once the right parameters are acquired, the patient can have the optimum results each time.

"All truth passes through three stages. First, it is ridiculed. Second, it is violently opposed. Third, it is accepted as being self-evident."

    Arthur Schopenhauer (1788-1860)

Chapter 3: The Q

    Once I learned about the effect of photomodulation on the meibomian glands, I began to experiment with different fluences and wavelengths. Intense Pulse Light will remain an in-office treatment performed by a doctor and never a treatment that patients can utilize at home because, if not administered properly, carries side effects. One report demonstrated that a doctor who utilized IPL without eye protection caused inflammation to the eyes. Theoretically, if IPL is used directly on the eye, the pigment of the retina could absorb it and cause problems. I looked at different wavelengths that would not cause harm to the eye, if used inappropriately.

    Currently, many wavelengths are used in healthcare to treat disease without side effects to the eyes. For example, red light has been used for facial rejuvenation. Blue light is used to help newborn infants recover from bilirubinemia and for acne. Surgeons and trainers utilize infrared to speed recovery for surgery and competitive sports. We tried all these different lights separately and in combination to see if any of these could be utilized to help the meibomian glands.

    We have spent the last 6 years studying the effects of light emitting diodes, LED, on MGD and DED. We demonstrated improvement in the signs and symptoms of DED with the use of a specific wavelength and power. Unlike IPL, the LED does not pulse, and you do not have to wait weeks between treatments. The patient applies the treatment at least twice a week to the lid margins (Figure 7). The power applied to the lids is less than what you achieve with IPL, and we found the effect to be less than what we achieved with IPL. I presented our results at the 2015 and 2016 American Society of Cataract and Refractive Surgery Annual Research Meeting.

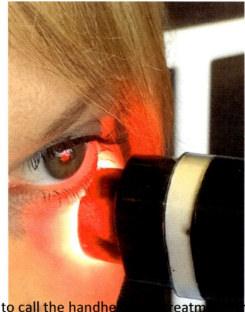

We began to call the handheld LED treatment the Quantum. After a while, the patients started calling it The Q for short. The Q is best used as an adjunct to IPL in moderate to severe MGD Dry Eye patients. In these patients, we complete the IPL protocol, and then, we allow the patient to utilize The Q at home. We find that the patient will not need as frequent maintenance IPL treatments with utilization of The Q. We also found that patients with mild DED can benefit from its use. Patients that are Fitzpatrick Skin Type 5 and 6 cannot have IPL and can utilize The Q to help. We feel that IPL is the best warm compress available, but the Q raises the temperature of the glands to help melt the abnormal thickened meibum. We have been able to apply The Q and express the glands in the clinic. We look forward to continuing our work on this new light technology.

"Unless we put medical freedom into the constitution the time will come when medicine will organize itself into an undercover dictatorship."

    Dr. Benjamin Rush (1746-1813)

Chapter 4: Diet & Supplements

The Ultimate Dry Eye Disease Diet

    During a busy clinic day, I never have time to go in-depth on what constitutes the ultimate DED Diet. Most patients have done a literature search and found out some of the basics in foods and supplements that can help them produce a better tear and reduce inflammation. If you accept that DED is a skin and gland problem causing poor a tear film, then any diet for your skin will help. You take a good skin diet and add some foods and supplements that have helped dry eye patients, and you have the ultimate DED diet. What is often skipped is what foods not to eat, which can be just as important. Before I give you my info, let me tell you that I try to live what I preach, but every once and awhile, I jones for some chips, fries, and key lime pie (say the last part with your best southern accent.) So I will not advise you to adopt a diet that is unrealistic. Incorporate the foods and supplements that you can and transition out the foods that are bad for you. If you need to cheat every once and awhile to stay sane, then go ahead and state it is for emotional support. I had a fitness trainer tell me one time that he eats things that he shouldn't every once and while just to stress out his digestive system so it wouldn't get lazy. I nodded my head and had a bite of key lime pie.

    One of the key essential nutrients your body needs to stay healthy, young, and vibrant is choline. Choline can be synthesized in small amounts by our bodies, but our diets need to supply much of it for normal functioning. Our body metabolizes the choline to produce phospholipids, like Phosphatidylcholine (PC). PC is found in our cell membranes. In a young child, 90 percent of our cell membrane is made up of PC. The cell membranes can be thought of as the protective walls of our cells that stop bad stuff from getting in and let good chemicals into the cells. If we do not ingest enough choline or our bodies have trouble making PC, then our cell membranes replace PC with hard fats and cholesterol. PC is used to make Very Low Density Lipoproteins, VLDL, a transport molecule that removes bad fatty acids from cells. A lack of choline can lead to non-alcoholic fatty liver disease. Choline, along with several B vitamins like B12, B6, folate, and riboflavin, is needed for the production of amino acids, nucleic acids, and S-adenosylmethione (SAMe). Our cells and glands that produce our own natural tear depend on the normal production of PC. I am surprised how a number of my patients are not eating a balanced diet. They are trying many specialized diets like gluten free, low carb, etc. but not eating the foods that can help their overall health and DED.

      Before you purchase PC from your neighborhood vitamin store, realize that the vitamin and supplement market is not as regulated as drugs are by the Food and Drug Administration, FDA. Dietary supplements must be manufactured under the current law put in place called Good Manufacturing Practices by the Dietary Supplement Health and Education Act (DSHEA). The manufacturer must register each facility with the FDA. Health claims concerning vitamins and supplements need documented proof. All these safeguards sound like enough, but what often happens is the National Institute of Health, NIH, publishes their funded study on a vitamin and then the manufacturers use their study to gain approval of their manufactured vitamin. Often times the quality of the supplement does not match the quality of the NIH study supplement, but manufacturer can make the same claim. Someone can shop for a supplement that they read about in a magazine that cited a NIH study, but the vitamin could have been manufactured in a different way, changing the bioavailability, absorption, and tolerability. Patients cannot find information about certain vitamins and supplements easily.

PC can be manufactured as Lecithin, and as long as the pill has 30% PC, it has the ability to call itself PC on the label. PC supplements will contain less than 20% choline. Manufacturers derive PC (often in the form of Lecithin) from egg yolk or soybeans. The soybean PC lecithin contains more polyunsaturated fatty acids (PUFAs), which has been shown to improve cardiovascular health, than egg yolks. Good food sources of Choline with large amount of PUFAs and will also help dry eye include but not limited to Salmon, Walnuts, Almonds, Scallop, Cod, Brussels Sprouts, Broccoli, Spinach, Cauliflower, Asparagus, and Milk Chocolate. There are other foods with high amount of Choline, like egg yolks, beef, animal liver, wheat germ, milk, peanut butter, flax seed, etc., but we are not building an overall diet, we are building one for DED. I am looking for foods that can check off many important components on our list without aggravating the inflammatory component of DED. For example, red meat contains a high amount of choline but also contains a pro inflammatory precursor, Arachidonic Acid. Another example would be egg yolk, shellfish, and whole milk products contain a high amount of choline but also contains cholesterol. Elevated levels of cholesterol in the body can cause atherosclerosis.

Milk can be as controversial as wheat products. We know that some people lack lactase, the enzyme needed to breakdown milk. Also, milk, especially skim milk, has a high glycemic index. Milk contains arachidonic acid, a pro-inflammatory compound that can be broken down into inflammatory mediators. Whole milk and dairy products, like butter, cheese, and ice cream, contain saturated fats creating problems like diabetes, obesity, and atherosclerosis. An alternative to milk would be almond milk.

If you need to cook some of these foods, reach for the Extra Virgin Olive Oil (EVOO) containing 98% to 99% triglycerides. The main fatty acids in EVOO are monounsaturates (oleic acid) with some saturates and PUFAs[14]. In the other one percent of EVOO, it contains the antioxidant Polyphenol, helping to fight the unstable atoms in our body that can damage the proteins, cells, and DNA called free radicals. We produce free radicals with normal biological processes in our body or introduce them into our body from pollutants like tobacco smoke. Patients who consume more EVOO have a lower risk of skin, breast, and colon cancers[15]. Oleic Acid has anti-inflammatory properties, aiding in the inflammatory component of DED and can be found in avocados and nuts.

Cooked tomatoes (better than raw) contain a high amount of the antioxidants lycopene and Zeaxanthin. Tomatoes protect against prostate cancer and acts as a natural sunscreen, helping to prevent skin cancers. The high potassium content helps control heart rate. It contains Vitamin A, flavonoid B complex, thiamine, folates, and niacin; all of these vitamins help the skin and eyes.

As a dessert, you can have a small bite of chocolate that contains cocoa flavonoids, a powerful antioxidant. Milk chocolate will give you some choline with some of the flavonoids. Dark chocolate contains the highest amount of flavonoids producing a decrease in cholesterol and risk of cardiovascular disease, an increase in sun protection and hydration to the skin, and increase blood flow to the brain. Don't forget that chocolate contains some caffeine. A study published in the journal Ophthalmology demonstrated that for some people caffeine increase tear production[16].

In what drinks will you consume your caffeine? How about drinking green tea containing antioxidants and catechins, like EGCG, bringing increased blood flow and oxygen to the face? A 2011 Journal of Nutrition stated that patients on green tea that contained polyphenols exhibited more elastic skin and less sun damage than the control.

I am often asked if a DED patient can have whole grains. Whole grains are better than processed starches but will raise your blood sugar (high glycemic index). A few DED patients may have a gluten allergy, and it is best to eliminate all possible allergens when combating DED. Whole wheat contains some choline, but I have shown a list of other foods that can provide you with choline and other beneficial nutrients. You can put whole grains in the not bad but no need to go out of your way to add them to your diet category.

If the Popeye cartoon were created today, the central food to give him strength would be kale, not spinach.   Don't misunderstand me, spinach is still a great vegetable, but kale provides more for the DED patient and can be found in just about any supermarket and that it is hard to pass up. Kale is one of the best sources of the powerful antioxidants lutein and zeaxanthin. I used to give baseball players supplements containing these nutrients to improve their night vision and cut down on glare. Lutein and Zeaxanthin reduces the free radicals produced in the skin by the sun. One cup of Kale provides you with over 100% of the daily requirement of Vitamin C and A.

I think all of the do and don't nutritional diets advise on **adequate water intake.** An adequate intake of water is essential in your DED diet. Your life depends on water because it is needed to carry nutrients into your cells and toxins out. Our bodies are largely made up of water, and we need to replace the water that we lose through the skin, urinary tract, gastrointestinal tract, and other systems, such as tear production. We often think of increasing our water intake by drinking a glass of water, but also think about eating more foods with high water content, like fruits and vegetables.

One of the problems that we have in modern society is that many of the over the counter medications and liquids we ingest are diuretics. Coffee, soft drinks, and alcohol are diuretics, causing dehydration when we drink these liquids. Always follow up by drinking a glass of water when you have coffee or alcohol. Replace your soft drink with water, and you can add a powdered vitamin supplement for flavor. Medications, such as antihistamines, will cause dehydration. Patients who are on any medication should increase their water intake to help flush any byproduct toxins that are produced in the body from the medication. Drink filtered or natural spring water instead of tap water because in several tests, tap water contains traces of hormones that can affect your tear production. Also, certain soft plastic water bottle containers are made with phthalates, an endocrine disruptor.

Phthalates can interfere with normal hormone production. Not only are phthalates used in water bottles but also in certain dairy products, cosmetics, shampoo, perfumes, and pesticides (always wash your fruits and vegetables). Phthalates have been shown to affect several hormone dependent processes like child development. Also found in certain plastic containers is bisphenol A, BPA. BPA has been linked to high blood pressure, prostate diseases, and brain development. BPA can also be use to coat the lining of canned foods. It is thought that in small amounts Phthalates and BPA are safe, but there are things you can do to lower your exposure. Cut back on canned foods, stay away from soft plastic water bottles, don't microwave plastics when heating your food, store food in glass instead of plastic containers, avoid plastics with recycling codes 3 and 7 because they may contain phthalates and BPA, avoid manufactured fragrances, eat and drink organic dairy products, and filter your water at home.

Supplements

Omega 3's have become the gold standard when talking about improving DED with diet and supplements. Omega 3's are polyunsaturated fatty acids (PUFAs) containing a special carbon group called omega because it rests of the end of the chain. There are 3 types of Omega 3's: alpha linolenic acid, ALA (in plants), eciosapentaenoic acid, EPA, and docosahexaenoic acid DHA (in fish).   Humans cannot produce full chain Omega 3, needing diet to manufacture longer chain fatty acids.   EPA and DHA has been shown to reduce inflammation. Studies have shown improvement in heart disease and arthritis.   Several studies, including an extensive study conducted by Dr. Penny Asbell, have shown supplementation with Omega 3's improve the signs and symptoms of DED. I have witnessed improvement in meibum of patients that increase Omega 3 in the their diet and with supplements. The Omega 3 fatty acids may provide improvement to the phospholipids of the meibum. With patients with MGD, the meibum becomes less like oil and more like toothpaste. Normal meibum has a melting point up to 32 degrees Celcius. Abnormal meibum has an increased melting point much higher than our body temperature of 37 degrees Celcius. It may be that the Omega 3's improve the lipids and decrease the melting points. I have never seen Omega 3 intake completely reverse abnormal MGD but it can help. Patients can eat salmon and sardines to increase their EPA and DHA. Atlantic Salmon contains the highest amount of Omega 3 with 2 grams per 100 grams. A small amount of EPA is made from ALA. Walnuts can be a good source of ALA.   I believe diet is the best way to achieve adequate amounts of Omega 3. You can also look to the Japanese diet[20] that has a high rate of fish intake which may explain their low rate of obesity, fat related cancers, and colon cancer. Since the American diet is different than the Japanese diet, I recommend the right fish oil supplements.

      The vast Omega 3 supplement market makes it difficult for patients to find the one that will provide the most benefit.   Since the market is loosely regulated, patients have to be careful in choosing an Omega supplement.   The Omega 3 supplements come in two forms: the Triglyceride and Ethyl Ester. The Triglyceride form resembles the natural form and is more expensive to manufacture. The Ethyl Ester can only be produced in a lab and is less expensive to produce. The easiest way to think of the difference is that ethyl ester is an alcohol based supplement.   The body requires more time to metabolize the alcohol based Omega 3. Studies have shown that the ethyl ester has less absorption and bioavailability than the triglyceride form[19]. One study showed over a 300% better absorption of the triglyceride compared to ethyl ester. Researchers have the ability to measure the amount of EPA and DHA levels charting the findings in an Omega 3 index. Researchers have shown a 25% difference in the Omega 3 index between triglyceride and ethyl ester.

You can use the Styrofoam cup test to determine if what type of Omega 3 you are currently taking. Puncture your capsule and place the oil on the Styrofoam cup. If the oil dissolves the cup in minutes then it is in the alcohol form; the ethyl ester can dissolve the bonds of the Styrofoam.

"One of the first duties of the physician is to educate the masses not to take medicine."

    Sir William Osler (1849-1919)

Chapter 5: Drop therapy: Non-medicated and Medicated

Artificial Tears

What's in a name?

    I think these drops are misnamed. There is no drop that can replace your natural tear because it contains protein, water, fat, mediators, anti-microbial products, and more. Our tear is designed to stay on your eye for a certain amount of time before it drains into the nasolacrimal drainage system (Figure 8). The lids contain an opening in each inner corner called the punctum, where the natural tear collects and dumps into the cannaliculi eventually going into the nasal sinus. Our anatomy is so perfect that it utilizes the tear in its entirety by having it lubricate our sinuses, so our nose does not dry out. We see this phenomenon all the time when we express the abnormal meibum from patients with MGD. When it drains into the sinuses, they feel like they have to sneeze because the abnormal meibum irritates the sinuses to the point that they have to blow their nose.

Figure 8. Nasolacrimal Drainage System (Can Stock Photo)

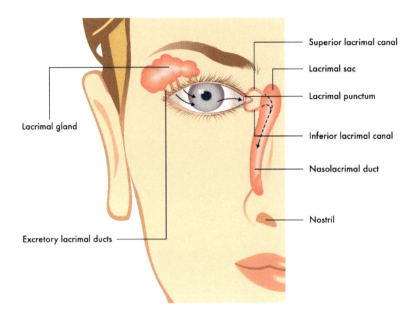

So there is no artificial tear that can replace our own healthy tear. We should call all these drops lubricants (Figure 9). In the severe cases of DED, patients need to use these lubricants continuously to wash away all the inflammatory mediators that are in their diseased tear. Now, I simply divide lubricants into two camps: 1. Medication 2. Non-Medication. The medicated lubricants have antimicrobial or anti-inflammatory properties. Some of these drops have strong scientific basis, and others do not. The non-medicated lubricants simply bath the eye with a gel, solution, or emulsion.

Figure 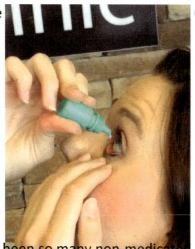 Clinic)

    There have been so many non-medicated lubricants with various claims that I could write a whole book on them, but the title of this book is not treatment now but in the future. These drops cannot not treat your dry eye but can only give you very temporary relief because all drops, even your own natural tear, eventually will work its way to the punctum and down the nasal lacrimal drainage system. Artificial tears help because they can clear the eye of inflammatory mediators by overwhelming them and eventually washing them away. If you have dry spots on the cornea, they can briefly coat the cornea so when you blink, you will not feel the dry spot. The tear can briefly correct the osmolarity of the eye. In dry eye patients, the tear osmolarity is increased, which could lead to pain.   A lubricant can not only change the osmolarity, but it can change the pH of the tear environment. Usually our tear will have a pH of 7.2, and our eye feels the best at this pH. In patients with DED, the pH is not normal. I have recorded more acidic and basic pHs in DED patients, but I have rarely recorded a normal pH.

    The abnormal pH plays an important role in why some patients prefer one lubricant than another.   Also, some patients tolerate some medications, and others do not. I learned early on that I could not recommend the same artificial tear to all patients. You will never have a one size fits all artificial tear for DED patients. Some doctor's mistakenly think that you match the artificial tear to the patient's type of dry eye disease. If the patient has MGD, then you give them a lubricant that is oiled based or gel-like. If they have Sjogren's disease, then you will give them a thinner water based lubricant. The lubricant rarely fits the disease. If you look at these drops as comfort drops and not as treatment, then your pick for the patient becomes trial and error, which I have learned is how patients have picked their drops. I have seen some drops preferred more often by my patients than others, but I always begin with preservative free lubricants because you eliminate a potential problem of allergy.

The most common preservative placed in ophthalmic drops is Benzalkonium chloride, BAK. We have seen that many patients have an allergic reaction to BAK. Corneal toxicity is also common with BAK. Some of the same inflammatory mediators are released in allergy as in DED, so a patient could be worsening their condition. Newer preservatives are being utilized for some drops now, but I have seen allergic reactions to the newer preservatives as well. If you find a drop that you love that has preservative, make sure that your doctor checks for toxicity, but my recommendation would be to continue looking until you find a preservative free lubricant. Also, I encourage my patients that are receiving treatment for DED to use the drop less because we want your own natural tear to work for you and washing it away with a lubricant defeats the purpose.

More than lubricants are the DED medications and lubricants that may have some medicinal benefits. I will cover these one by one. I will also cover some drops that are not on the market yet but could be by the year 2020.

We have to start with Restasis because it was the first drop to receive FDA approval as a DED drop. As a referral DED center, most of my patients have been prescribed Restasis at some point in their journey to improvement. I utilized cyclosporine drops before FDA approval because I understood the inflammatory component of DED and knew that decreasing T cells (inflammatory mediator decreased with the use of Restasis) would help the symptoms. I consider DED to be an inflammatory disease so having an anti-inflammatory on board will improve the ocular environment. Restasis is preservative free, so it fulfills my criteria for acceptable lubricant. What Restasis is not is a treatment. I have never seen Restasis improve meibomian gland dysfunction. I have seen minimal improvements of tear film of patients who have been on Restasis for over a 3 month period. Many patients complain about Restasis as a lubricant, and it is probably because they cannot tolerate the pH of the drop. When patients on Restasis begin treatment in our clinic, I usually wean them off the medication. I actually try to encourage them to taper all drops.

Tacrolimus[28], also known as FK506, is an immunosuppressant with a similar mechanism of action as Restasis, cyclosporine A. It can be 100 times more potent than cyclosporine A[29] and has been used in dogs for dry eye. We have used it in patients with severe eye allergies because it also prevents histamine release from mast cells. It is a macrolide natural compound, like the one used for the antibiotic Erythromycin. (Some doctors have tried using Oral Erythromycin to decrease the skin inflammation associated with Rosacea, MGD, and DED.) Tacrolimus inhibits calcineurin, decreasing T-cell function. The mechanism of action not only stops the T-cells but other inflammatory mediators, like interleukins.

Lifitegrast is a topical anti-inflammatory medication that is awaiting FDA approval. The medication binds to a cell surface protein, LFA1- lymphocyte function-associated antigen-1, preventing the binding of T-cells to Intercellular Adhesion Molecule 1 – ICAM 1. Simply put, before T-cells can be incorporated into the cells to release and recruit inflammatory mediators, Lifitegrast blocks the cells they need to infiltrate the tissues.

Amniotic membranes have been used to help heal damaged corneas due to injury or infection. A membrane can provide stem cells to the cornea that can differentiate and provide normal cells for repair. The epithelial cells on the surface of the cornea are regenerating every 3 to 5 days. The effect of the membrane helps during the 7 days that it stays on the eye. The effects are temporary because the membrane dissolves, and the cells continue to regenerate. Researchers have been working on providing the positive benefits of the amnion but for a longer and more consistent basis. A company is now utilizing Human Amniotic Fluid (HAF), the fluid the surrounds the fetus and is in continuous contact to the child, as an eye drop. The amniotic fluid contains a higher concentration of growth factors than the membrane, (Epidermal Growth Factor, Tissue Growth Factor – Beta, Fibronectin). HAF is spun down like you would with blood to extract serum. The company processes the amniotic serum to make a new topical medication.

   Umbilical Cord Blood Serum (UCBS), has also been used as eye drops. The UCBS is collected from the umbilical vein of the placenta after delivery of the baby. Usually you can obtain 40mLs of serum from one cord blood sample. Cord blood has been shown to have higher concentrations of certain growth factors than adult blood serum. We are currently finding better ways to separate out the unwanted portions of the blood and concentrate the beneficial factors that can reduce infection, promote healing, and relieve the symptoms of DED.

   One company has been utilizing human platelets from young healthy donors to produce a platelet rich source of topical eye drops. Similar to autologous PRP, the company removes the clotting factors and other unwanted products of the blood, leaving the beneficial factors. All these non-autologous products will have to prove purity, so that patients can administer the drop safely.

   Recently, we have been studying a drop that we discovered when we were training dry eye specialists in Australia. Oculocin Propo is a new natural eye drop that is utilized to treat the symptoms of conjunctivitis (inflammation of the outer layer of the eye) and Dry Eye Disease. The key ingredients in Oculocin are Propolis, Aloe Vera, and Chamomilla. You may have heard of these ingredients in other familiar products. So, my first concern was does this drop sting? It is the exact opposite; all the patients that we tried Oculocin on stated that the drop felt great on contact. One reason may be that Oculocin is preservative free and comes in sterile vials. In a limited test of 20 dry eye patients, we had no allergic reactions, stinging, or burning.

How will it help DED? I believe that the active ingredients in Oculocin need more studies, but we do know that studies have shown that Propolis is a resin-like substance found in plants. Actually, bees take this resin from plants back to their hives to coat their hives. (Does the resin coat the ocular surface?) We know that Propolis has antibacterial and antifungal properties to protect the plant. (Can Propolis fight the lid infection (Blepharitis)? A common sequelae of Dry Eye Disease.) It has been known for centuries that the plant based Aloe Vera and Chamomile have anti-inflammatory properties. We documented that patients on Oculocin had decreased lid and eye inflammation. Patients reported that their eyes felt less irritated during the day with the administration of one drop of Oculocin.

Prostaglandins are one of the major inflammatory mediators that cause damage and pain to the eye. Early in the inflammatory cascade, phospholipids are converted by phospholipases to one of the precursors to prostaglandins. Topical steroids block phospholipases, preventing the conversion of phospholipids. Steroid drops extensively control inflammation but cause increase in eye pressure, cataracts, susceptibility to infection, and in some patients, may cause personality changes. There are several types of topical steroids out in the market that have different potencies and effectiveness. Steroids control the inflammation of DED and help with symptoms. You can use topical steroids for a few days in DED, but much longer, you run the risk of complications. Steroids will not be a viable option in DED until the side effects can be minimized or eliminated.

Topical non-steroidal anti-inflammatory drugs, NSAIDs,

control inflammation by a different mechanism. The enzyme cyclo-oxygenase, COX, is used to finish the conversion of phospholipids to prostaglandins. NSAIDs blocks COX, stopping the production of inflammatory mediators. NSAIDs have less of a side effect profile than steroids but also carry less potency. We presented our research showing that dry eye patients demonstrated no complications with the long term use of NSAIDs to control inflammation and DED symptoms at the Johns Hopkins Current Concepts in Ophthalmology meeting several years ago. There are published reports that generic and older generation topical NSAIDs can cause deterioration of the cornea (corneal melts). One report stated that patients with DED are more susceptible to corneal melts. We showed that the published report assumed that patients with plugs suffered from DED and that it was a risk factor for melts. We have successfully used topical NSAIDs to control symptoms of dry eye.

You will be hearing the term biologics in terms of improving the signs and symptoms of disease. Any drug produced by a biological system as opposed to being manufactured in a lab is called a biologic. Some common examples of biologics are Human Growth Hormone and Insulin. You hear advertisements for biologics everyday on TV when you see a commercial for Humira or Enbrel. Most of these biologics decrease the inflammatory cytokine, Tumor Necrosis Factor Alpha. Pharmaceutical companies are now converting some of these oral biologics to topical drops to control inflammation. We have been involved in studies to control intraocular inflammation with biologics with favorable effects when compared to topical steroids, without the downsides. A drawback is biologics are more expensive and difficult to produce. Also, the body may recognize the biologic as foreign and send antibodies to eradicate the medication. We currently do not understand the full effect and side effect profile of topical biologics.

Researchers are studying the effectiveness of biologics for dry eye disease. Physicians at Harvard Medical School demonstrated that the topical use of Anakinra[17], a recombinant of

Interluekin -1Ra, a biologic that is approved for the treatment of Rheumatoid Arthritis. We sent some of our patients for treatment with Kineret drops with mixed results. In a randomized study conducted by Harvard, the topical drops improved the signs and symptoms of DED as compared to artificial tears. Biologics could replace topical steroids and NSAIDs as the topical anti-inflammatory of choice in cases of DED with uncontrolled inflammation. I think we are early in the research for biologics, but by the year 2020, we may find a biologic that is more specific for the inflammation caused by DED.

    The concept utilizing autologous blood serum to heal eye disease is several decades old. Dr. Fox et al. published a paper in 1984 in on the Beneficial Effect of Artificial Tears made with autologous serum in patients with Keratoconjunctivitis Sicca[10]. Dr. Tsubota et al published a paper on the treatment of dry eye by autologous serum application in Sjogren's Syndrome[11] and has been championing the treatment ever since. I have heard many tales on how the concept became a universal practice. In the early days (late 1990's) of Lasik, it was seen that these patients developed a transient dry eye that would last a few weeks and eventually would resolve. Back then, we would use an instrument to construct a flap on the cornea, similar to a book cover, that we would lift revealing the stroma of the cornea. We would laser the stroma to achieve the correction to the refractive error of the patient and then lay the flap back down, protecting our surgery. The patient would go home and let the flap heal with their eyes closed. The next morning the flap was sealed, and the patient had achieved their desired correction. The technology that created the flap, microkeratome, would go onto the eye and create suction on the eye that would keep the eye in position as the blade would construct the flap. We believed that the suction created by the microkeratome paralyzed the goblet cells, causing an imbalance in the tear film. The poor tear film would leave the patient with dry eye and decreased vision. Sometimes, the blade would not only cut the cornea, but it would also cut blood vessels on the conjunctiva and, rarely, the lid. The cutting of the blood vessels was not noticed by the patient to any extent, but what the surgeon noticed at post op is the patients that had a bloody Lasik procedure did not have the dry eye as a post-operative complication.

In 1998, I graduated at the perfect time to be a Lasik surgeon. The procedure in 1998 was about to have its best years in terms of numbers because it was a new successful procedure that finally could offer patients a sophisticated way of becoming independent of glasses and contacts. I moved to Tennessee and became the first Lasik Surgeon in the state. I had trained with some of the pioneers of the procedure including Dr. Kerry Assil and Dr. Steve Brint. Because of this, I felt comfortable becoming one of the top Lasik surgeons in the country. It seemed everyone was having Lasik at that time. I had my Lasik procedure in 1999. In the early years, I would complete over a 1000 patients a year. The good thing about so much volume in a short period of time is you can see trends quickly. I experienced the decrease in dry eye signs and symptoms of patients who had bleeding with their Lasik procedure. It was determined that our blood contained many helpful mediators that assist in wound healing.

Many doctors hypothesized that we could extract blood from a dry eye patient and spin it down to obtain the serum, utilizing it as a dry eye ocular medication. You must remember that the field of Dry Eye was in its infancy. In fact, it was not a disease but a syndrome back then. If a day of serum could help a Lasik patient overcome post-operative dry eye, then sustained exposure to blood serum could fix dry eye. Of course, we now know that Dry Eye is a disease like any other and that a medication, no matter how good, could only help manage the disease. We began giving our DED patients their serum in drop form four times a day. Some patients felt relief, but others did not. The treatment never solved the problem of treating MGD, but some patients felt some relief from the drops. Also, autologous blood serum has been used to help heal the cornea in certain diseases.

Where autologous blood serum is gaining ground is in the healing of the corneal nerves. The corneal nerves are responsible for the sensations of touch, pain, and temperature. They also play a role in the blink reflex, wound healing, and tear production. Proper function of the front surface of the eye is dependent on our tears and the cornea. It has been shown many diseases can harm the cornea nerves so that feeling can be lost, leading to destruction of the front surface of the eye. Studies have shown Lasik in the environment of dry eye can lead to abnormal regeneration of the nerves after flap creation and healing, leading to worsening symptoms[12]. (The reason that we perform a surface ablation, epilasik, if patients have any signs and symptoms of dry eye. We cover Lasik in Dry Eye later in the book.) We have also seen that longstanding inflammation from dry eye disease can affect the cornea nerves as well.

We can now look at the morphology of the corneal nerves by direct observation by confocal microscopy. Dr. Matsumoto was one of the first to show that autologous serum could be used to help people with cornea nerve damage, neurotrophic keratopathy. For the last two years, we have had doctors present data showing that autologous serum can improve the cornea nerve architecture when studied by confocal microscopy. The neuro-regenerative effects of blood serum are now accepted. We have been utilizing autologous serum not to improve MGD but to help patients with corneal nerve pain. We treat the underlying cause of their dry eye disease. For example, with a patient with MGD DED, we treat with IPL, and if they are still having nerve pain with no signs and symptoms of DED, we treat them with autologous serum.

What will you get from autologous serum? Nerve Growth Factor, NGF, is a vital component in the regeneration of damaged nerves and normal maintenance. In injury to the cornea, whether from inflammation, trauma, or Lasik, requires NGF to repair itself. NGF may have some antimicrobial properties as well to prevent infection after injury. Vascular Endothelial Growth Factor, VEGF, also has neuroprotective capability. As I stated before, we have an alphabet soup of mediators that function for normal function of the eye, but NGF and VEGF have been studied the most. Autologous blood serum contains many factors, including NGF and VEGF. Most physicians will centrifuge the patient's blood and then dilute the drop in various ratios and different vehicles (artificial tears, balanced salt solution, or straight without any additives). We have tried all different combinations presented in the literature. We have been impressed with the response, but we have started to use a new form of blood treatment called Platelet Rich Plasma, PRP.

Research has found that using Umbilical Cord Serum eye drops may be more effective than blood serum because the higher concentration of beneficial mediators. It could be that attaining a higher concentration of the bioactive mediators may improve the efficacy of serum treatment. PRP may be the best way to concentrate active factors while removing useless components of the blood. In the standard serum procedure, the red blood cells are spun down to the bottom, and you are left with the rest of the serum. In PRP, we are able to extract the platelets that have Platelet Derived Growth Factor (PDGF), TGF-B, VEGF, Sema7A, and NGF in the form of Brain Derived Neurotrophic Factor (BDNF).

We are currently using the PRP[13] (Figure 10) system where blood is collected and anticoagulated with citrate, followed by centrifugation to separate the PRP. The red blood cells and platelet poor plasma is removed to render a highly concentrated form of PRP. We are achieving levels up to 14 times greater than if we were conducting simple blood serum drop collection without the PRP system. We mix the PRP with our own vehicle and have the patient utilize the drop two to four times a day. One bottle is used per month with the other four bottles frozen until time of use. We have found quicker wound healing utilizing PRP for corneal injury. DED patients report increase comfort in PRP as opposed to plain serum drops. PRP has become the preferred autologous blood product in other specialties, such as Neurosurgery, Orthopedics, and Plastic Surgery, and I believe it will be the preferred modality in Ophthalmology.

Figure 10. PRP (Toyos Clinic)

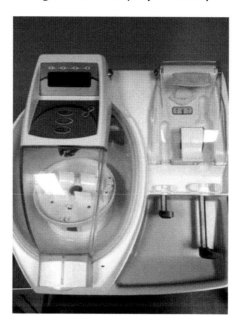

Honey is one treatment that has been used since ancient times and may be a treatment in DED. Honey is a sugar solution derived from nectar, gathered and modified by the honeybee. Studies by Albietz et. al. showed that the use of a specific honey[21] could reduce the amount of lipase creating bacteria on the skin. They used Leptospermum shrub honey called Manuka, a stable honey used in several medical research studies. A company in Australia, a country rich in Leptospermum, produces a honey-based eye drop called Optimel. We are currently conducting studies with our patients utilizing Optimel with promising results. I find the viscous nature of the purified honey to last on the eye longer than normal lubricant drops and provide some short term relief. We would like to see the long term effects of applying Optimel on the skin, lid margin, and lashes to observe the effects as a cleanser. Optimel contains preservatives that lower the pH of solution, causing some stinging to patients when first applied.

The mode of delivering medical and non-medical lubricants may change over time. Instead of a drop, we could use a delivery system inserted in the fornix. Lacrisert is a once-daily slow release insert of hydroxypropyl cellulose. The same system could be used for medications so that patients would not have to worry about putting drops in the eye all day. Companies have also experimented with placing a miniature insert in the nasolacrimal duct that would release medicine to the eye.

Electrical stimulation has been tried in many ways for many diseases. Who can forget the use of electric shock therapy to treat schizophrenia? Or the use of electric paddles to stimulate a stopped heart? Researchers at Stanford University are working on an implantable miniature electrical technology to stimulate the lacrimal gland to secrete more water. Another company is working on approval of an electrical device inserted up the nostrils delivering shock to increase tear production. I never dismiss an idea, but I believe electric shock therapy may be a step back as compared to the sophistication of light therapy. If we use NASA research as a guide, we see that they are not applying electrical stimulation to the astronauts for better physical function but light therapy. We will keep an open mind and follow the progress.

"He is the best physician who is the most ingenious inspirer of hope."

    Samuel Taylor Coleridge (1772-1834)

Chapter 6: Pain

    I always ask DED patients what is their number one complaint. Some common answers are dryness, redness, scratchiness, and poor vision; the list goes on. Some patients state that their eyes hurt all the time. I rotated through an orthopedic pain clinic as a medical student. The patients that complain about DED pain remind me of the chronic back pain patients. The DED patients state that they feel a constant ache that does not go away with drops. I have been able to help several of these patients with IPL, the Q, PRP, and Autologous Serum drops, but we have some patients that have improvement in their disease but still have pain. We have tried several different treatments with varying degrees of success. Please exhaust all treatments for the underlying disease before you try the outliers described here.

    A group of Lasik patients complain of post-operative eye pain. Most of these patients have undiagnosed DED prior to their surgery, and then the Lasik can exacerbate the problems due to poor healing of the corneal nerves. The reason that DED is missed is one of the treatments for pain. Many Lasik patients are soft contact lens wearers, and we find that the contact lens can mask the symptoms of dry eye by anesthetizing the eye by pressing on the corneal nerves and providing a barrier between the lids and the cornea. Once you remove the contact lens permanently, the patient can now "feel" their dry eye. Before surgery, we have the patient out of their contact lenses for a period of time. If we diagnose DED, then we have the patient stay out of their contact lenses longer. After these patients are out of their contacts, they begin to feel the symptoms that go along with their signs.

The Boston Foundation of Sight has taken the knowledge that contact lenses can control pain by manufacturing custom scleral lenses that can help these patients. They have developed the prosthetic replacement of the ocular surface ecosystem (PROSE) device. This is a scleral lens that forms a dome that they describe as a margarita glass shape over the cornea. The device is made of a gas permeable hard plastic that creates a space between the device and the cornea that is filled with sterile saline. Theoretically, the fluid stays in the space all day long until the patient removes the contact lens.

We have tried contact lenses and scleral lens for patients. Some patients have had relief of pain, if the underlying DED is controlled. Even in the patients that it has worked on, eventually have the pain returns because the anesthetic effect cannot last. Some patients complain that the scleral lens can be uncomfortable and hard to place on the eye. We always try a large contact lens first before we recommend spending the considerable amount of money on a customized lens. If they feel no relief with the contact lens, then we try not get their hopes up to high with PROSE, but when you are in pain, you will exhaust all available remedies.

We have also tried Pregabalin, Lyrica, in a few patients to control eye pain. **Lyrica is an antiepileptic drug, like Neurontin, or Gabapentin. It is approved for pain from diabetic neuropathy or post herpetic neuralgia in adults. These drugs bind to the alpha2-delta protein at the nerve endings causing decrease release of the neurotransmitters reducing pain. We have tried this with a handful of people with mixed results. We had one patient who felt that they had suicide ideation, one of the side effects with the drug, with little relief on his eye pain. We did eventually test this patient for a vitamin deficiency and discovered that he had B12 deficiency. These patients can be frustrating, especially if you improve their signs and symptoms of DED.**

Naltrexone has been used to block the effects of opioids for years. I never prescribe traditional pain meds for eye pain because I have seen the addictive nature of these medications. Low Dose Naltrexone[30] is a hot new topic because it has been shown in some studies to help with autoimmune conditions and pain. One study demonstrated a 30% decrease in pain symptoms in Fibromyalgia patients. In pain, glia cells are activated to produce inflammatory mediators. The LDN may block the glia cells from activating the inflammatory cascade. We have tried LDN in a handful of patients with no symptomatic effect.

"Good information is the best medicine."

Dr. Michael E. Debakey (1908-2008)

Chapter 7: Surgery

Conjunctivochalasis Surgery

In every other body part, we can accept the fact that longstanding inflammation will cause destructive changes that will change anatomy and prevent normal function, but when I talk to patients about this in the eye, they have a tough time accepting the concept. Longstanding DED will change the surfaces of the eye and lid. Patients with chronic DED for many years usually have changes to the conjunctiva that are noticeable. The conjunctiva can be grayish, red from injected blood vessels, and/or redundant. I have patients that complain more about the redness of their eyes than the pain from dry eye. I had one CEO of a company who stated he could deal with the scratchiness of blinking, but he was upset that people during business meetings would ask him if he slept enough the night before or some would joke that he was a marijuana smoker. The straight-laced CEO hated these comments.

Now, the bad appearance of DED is one thing, but the redundancy of the conjunctiva can cause functional problems. The conjunctiva appears wrinkled, and with each blink, you can see the excess conjunctiva come between the two lids coming together. The problem with an obstruction of blink is that we need the apposition of the lids to excrete the contents of the Meibomian Glands. I describe to patients that the worn out conjunctiva is like carpet that has been water logged for a long period of time. Eventually, the carpet becomes wrinkled and pulls off the floor. Now, you can dry out the carpet and hope that it retains its prior form, but more times than not, it never sits on the floor the same way. The conjunctiva with inflammation achieves the wrinkled carpet syndrome, pulling away from the sclera. So when the patient attempts to blink and push out the meibum, it doesn't happen because the conjunctiva gets in the way.

In some patients when you control the MGD and inflammation, the conjunctiva regains its normal appearance and function. Usually, I have seen recovery in young patients under the age of 50 who have had moderate disease for a few years. In our clinic, we see the worst cases of DED, so even with maximum therapy, the conjunctiva remains red, gray, and redundant. If you achieve enough improvement that the function improves to normal and the redness is reduced from a maximum 4 to barely perceivable 2, some patients state they are satisfied with the results and decline further options.

For patients that we cannot regain function, we offer them Conjunctivochalasis Surgery. There are several ways to attack the problem with surgery. We have tried all of the most popular surgeries. One type of surgery is to remove the extra conjunctiva inferiorly and sew in an amniotic graft. The surgery improves the redundancy, but in the incorporation of the graft, you can have an undesirable cosmetic appearance. Also, a common complication is that the graft will irritate the patient's eye, so they rub the eye, disrupting the healing and causing lid irritation. We have tried excising the excess conjunctiva inferiorly and allowed it to heal without sutures. The technique has a better effect than a graft but takes longer to heal than if sutures are used. Some surgeons close the conjunctiva after excision by cauterizing the ends together. Cautery works to close the wound but leaves some jagged edges that patients feel for a period time before eventually smoothing out. We found that removing the excess inferiorly with a special dissolvable suture reduces irritation.

Patients recover better function of their natural blink that aides in the secretion of meibum. We have shown improved TBUT times and symptomatology with the technique. Now, some patients are satisfied with the appearance, but others want more improvement in the appearance. When patients have excess sun exposure with DED, the conjunctiva not only becomes redundant but actually starts to lose its normal architecture, appearing raised and rough. We called this diseased conjunctiva a pinquecula when it does not encroach on to the cornea and a pterygium when it does. In both cases, even the slightest irritation will cause the abnormal tissue to inflame, looking even more unsightly. In the case of a pinquecula with concurrent conjuctivochalasis, I will remove the pinquecula and excess conjunctiva, helping the patient's function and appearance. The conjunctiva that is covered by the lower and upper lid when the eye is opened is not exposed to the elements and appears cosmetically better. Sometimes, I will utilize the normal appearing conjunctiva and create a graft to place the exposed area. In a pterygium excision, I will remove the abnormal tissue on the cornea as well as the abnormal and redundant conjunctiva.

    In some patients, you are concerned with inflammation after excision. Some surgeons utilize Mitomycin C, or MMC, an antimetabolite that prevents fibrosis after surgery. The original use for Mitomycin was in cancer patients to prevent growth of the cancer cells. We utilize Mitomycin in low doses to prevent scarring. For a typical conjunctivochalasis surgery, I do not use Mitomycin C because, like any medicine, it does have side effects. Sometimes, MMC can disrupt normal tissues, leading to thinning of the sclera, necessitating a graft to prevent a penetration of the posterior tissues. In pinquecula and pterygium excisions, I use low level MMC that is flushed from normal tissues with balance salt solution. I find the MMC prevents inflammation and recurrence.

    A treatment called Eye Brite made the rounds years ago after a Korean surgeon began removing all the conjunctiva of red eye patients that wanted a whiter looking eye. In the procedure, not only did the surgeon remove the conjunctiva but also applied MMC to achieve even a brighter looking eye. When it made its way to America, I happened to work in a clinic near the doctor that was performing the procedure, and I saw firsthand the bad side effects of the procedure. Logically, if you think about the procedure, you are removing the conjunctiva which contains the Goblet Cells, the protein producing cells for tears. The patients that I had the chance to treat post-Eye Brite procedure were having significant dry eye problems with an abnormal tear film. In the environment of a poor tear film and MMC, the patients were more prone to thinning of the sclera. We had a few patients that needed patch grafts to repair the sclera. Some surgeons have continued to perform the Eye Brite procedure because the eyes look better, but I do not recommend it to patients because the complications are too common and serious.

I find a modification to the Eye Brite procedure makes it a more viable procedure in the future. Patient with a pinquecula can have the abnormal conjunctiva removed safely because the goblet cells no longer exist in that area. Once removed, you utilize normal looking conjunctiva to cover the bare sclera at the place of removal, and you leave normal conjunctiva intact. We have fourth generation topical steroid drops that perform well in controlling the inflammation created with surgery. Now, some patients require MMC, even in the face of stronger topical steroids, but I usually reserve MMC for patients that have reoccurrence of the pinquecula from prior excision surgery. We have been able to achieve whiter appearing eyes without sacrificing the safety of the patient by scaling back greatly the original concept. I must admit that with the added safety you lose some degree of white appearance, but a little less shade of whiteness in the face of no complications is a tradeoff that I and my patients accept.

A concept that my wife, Melissa Toyos, MD, an Oculoplastic surgeon, discusses often is lid sagging effects on dry eye. As we age, the fibroblasts of the skin produce less and less collagen. Collagen is needed in the skin to help maintain the youthful structure and appearance. In a blink, we need enough rigidity in the skin to squeeze the meibomian glands and release meibum. Our fibroblasts stop producing collagen after the age of 28, but we have many available technologies and skin applications that stimulate our fibroblasts to produce collagen. Medical grade skin care lines contain antioxidants and other substances that the skin absorbs and stimulate fibroblasts, such as vitamin C, alpha hydroxys, retinoids to name a few. Intense Pulse Light and certain LED technologies stimulate collagen formation. Many doctors utilize Erbium and CO2 lasers to achieve more dramatic facial rejuvenation. Dr. Melissa Toyos performs a specific laser procedure that she has pioneered called the Mixto Laser Lift (Figure 11), using a special fractionated CO2 laser. She has seen that Mixto Laser Lift around the lids will tighten the lids and improve the normal blink apposition. After the procedure, the lid has a more normal surface for contraction to aid in the release of meibum. We have seen an increase in TBUT and improvement in DED symptoms with Mixto Laser Lift alone.

Figure 11. Before and After Mixto Laser Lift (Toyos Clinic)

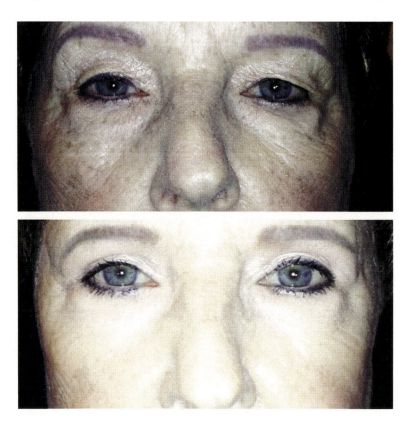

Some doctors advocate blinking exercises for their patients to improve meibum secretion, but if the problem is anatomical such as with Conjunctivochalsis or Dermatochalsis, then blinking harder and better will not solve the DED problem. You should not have to work harder on a natural reflex but treat the problem that decreases the production from your blink.

Can Dry Eye Patients have Lasik

Figure 12. Lasik Procedure (Toyos Clinic)

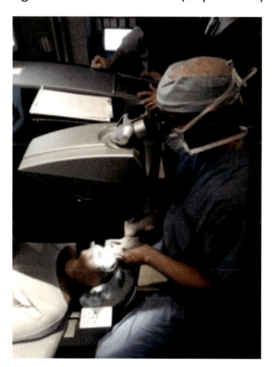

My first "Lasik" case ever was a PRK (photorefractive keratectomy) in 1996. PRK consisted of scraping the front surface of the eye with an eye spatula to clear the top part of the cornea, the epithelium, so that you could use the laser to reshape the central part of the cornea. The epithelium consists of cells that regenerate every week. Old epithelial cells slough off as new epithelium is made and replaces the old. This is why when you suffer a scratch of the cornea it heals with new cells in a few days.

The cornea is like a book that has sheets of collagen similar to sheets of paper. In PRK, you are scraping the cover of the book to reveal the pages and perform laser correction.   The problem with PRK is that the scraping and subsequent healing led to scarring and haze, precipitating poor vision due to halos and glare. PRK evolved to Lasik when blade technologies could produce a flap that consisted of epithelium and the collagen sheets that do not regenerate. We are essentially lifting the cover of the book for laser treatment, and then we would lay the cover back down, avoiding scraping and the haze problem. The technique evolved to laser technologies, instead of a blade, that could produce a flap. We currently utilize the latest of these laser flap creators called the Wavelight FS200 with Green Technology, producing a consistent reproducible flap every time that is centered on the pupil, but PRK-type procedures have not become obsolete because the prevalence of DED.

Some patients are not candidates for Lasik because they do not have enough pages in their book to create a flap (the cornea is not thick enough to produce a flap and have laser reshaping), have a corneal scar, or they have a dry eye. We have seen that in some dry eye patients, the making of a flap could cause an exacerbation of dry eye symptoms. The theory being that dry eye patients nerve architecture of the cornea does not heal properly after the procedure. The corneal nerves are responsible for pain sensation and the tear reflex for normal production. In dry eye patients, we avoid making a flap. The problem in performing PRK in any of these patients is that they are at higher risk of haze. The solution to the problem of PRK was solved over a decade ago with a technology called the Epilift, allowing us to perform Epilasik. In Epilasik, the technology lifts the outer sheet of epithelium without the trauma of scraping. The other advantage of the Epilift is that it gives you a uniform sheet of epithelium with smooth edges. PRK scraping is not uniform, and the edges are haphazard. We have been performing Epilasik successfully for 13 years. We presented a study of Epilasik versus Lasik. We performed Epilasik on one eye of a patient and Lasik on the other eye. There was no statistical difference in vision or reported halo and glare in the eyes after 3 months. The best thing about Epilasik is that you will not see the haze that is seen in PRK. The drawback of Epilasik is Lasik patients heal by the next day, but Epilasik needs about 4 days to completely heal the front surface.

In DED patients who desire Lasik, we perform Epilasik to not disrupt the corneal nerves. Epilasik has solved the problem of exacerbation of dry eye symptoms in dry eye patients. We caution all of our patients that the eyes will feel dry right after Lasik or Epilasik because the goblet cells on the conjunctiva decrease the production of mucin. The decrease of protein production to the tear causes irregular tears and symptoms. The goblet cells usually take a few weeks to resume normal function. All Lasik and Epilasik patients should plan on utilizing artificial tears after surgery until they recover a normal tear. DED patients can have Epilasik, but there was another procedure before Lasik that people choose to achieve freedom from glasses and contacts and that was RK.

RK and DED

During my residency in Ophthalmology, I watched a few Radial Keratotomy (Figure 13) procedures to correct near sightedness and astigmatism. The procedure consisted of blade cuts on through the epithelium and into the stroma. The deeper in to the stroma, the more effect you would achieve. The more radial cuts the more effect. Arcuate cuts on the cornea would help correct astigmatism. The cornea is normally like a sphere, and when radial cuts are applied, the center flattens. Our tear uses the round shape of the eye to distribute the tear equally throughout the eye. Just think if I put a drop of water on the top of a handball, the tear would spread from the center and roll down. When the cornea is flattened in the center in RK, it is like putting a drop on a flat table. Instead of equal distribution, you have a tear that sits in the center with very little movement. We see the tear in RK pool in the center, causing dry spots on various parts of the cornea where the tear has not traveled to after the blink. When a tear is not distributed equally, we see pooling of the tear to various parts. If you add arcuate incisions to the cornea, the irregularity becomes worse.

Figure 13. RK scars (Toyos Clinic)

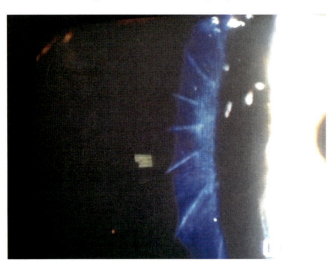

If the tear does not evenly distribute due to flattening of the cornea, the only possibility that a patient has available is Epilasik. I have seen the procedure improve the shape of the cornea without harming the corneal nerves. Some patients with arcuate incisions affect the nerves, complicating the problem even more. Some patients had several incision in different directions causing pain even after having Epilasik. In those patients, the only thing you can do to help them is Oculocin, PRP, or Optimel.

A New Procedure, A New Bit of Caution

We were correcting astigmatism in patients during cataract surgery with arcuate incisions created by a blade. The blade created arcuate incisions never achieved consistent results, but recently, lasers have been utilized in cataract surgery (Figure 14). The main use for most surgeons is laser arcuate incisions for astigmatism. The laser makes the creation of an arcuate incision more accurately, producing better results. However, a word of caution in DED patients, if the laser incisions are made to long, it can exacerbate dry eye symptoms, mimicking what we see in DED patients that undergo Lasik. In Cataract and Lasik surgery, the key for DED patients is to improve the ocular surface for improved results and choose the procedure that has the least chance to worsen their condition.

Figure 14. Laser Cataract Surgery patient (Toyos Clinic)

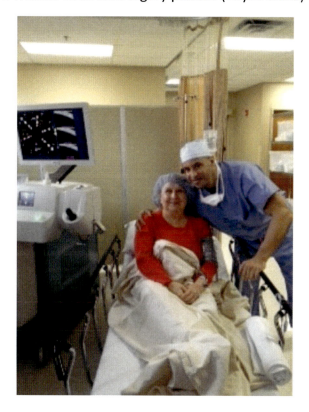

"What spirit is so empty and blind, that it cannot recognize the fact that foot is more noble than the shoe, and skin more beautiful than the garment with which it is clothed?"

    Michelangelo (1475-1564)

Chapter 8: Skin

Patients have often heard me say that DED is a skin and gland condition that affects the eyes. I have covered all the treatments for all the glands that help secrete the tear film, but I have only touched on the treatments for the skin when talking about Intense Pulse Light and The Q. I integrated aesthetics into my ophthalmology practice 16 years ago. At the time, it was uncommon for ophthalmologists to offer aesthetics. Now, it seems that every ophthalmologist has discovered the benefits of incorporating cosmetic procedures and surgery into their practice. My wife and I give countless lectures and seminars teaching ophthalmologists that the two specialties are a natural fit. The thinnest skin in the body is the lids, and no other doctor knows this area better. I have seen many plastic surgeons and dermatologists who will not operate on the lids because the skin is so different, and more importantly, they know that a surgery on the lids could affect eye function. If too much skin in the lid area is removed, then the patient cannot close their eyes or blink properly to release meibum. Other specialties understand the importance of the ophthalmologist's understanding of the skin, and now, we have to appreciate the importance of our knowledge. What I have learned in these years is that to ignore the skin as an ophthalmologist is to deprive our patients of the best treatment possible especially when it comes to DED.

Our skin (Figure 15) is a regenerative organ that renews itself every month. The top layer of your skin, the epidermis, is composed of dead skin cells that will eventually slough off, or you can choose to remove the layer with an aesthetic procedure, such as microdermabrasion. Patients love the look of their skin right after the periodic microdermabrasion or IPL. The middle layer of the skin is called the dermis and contains all of the structures, including glands, hair follicles, blood vessels, pigment cells (melanocytes), nerve fibers, and fibroblasts. The fibroblasts produce collagen and elastin. Collagen is the protein that makes up most of our skin. Elastin is what gives our skin elasticity to bounce back, without leaving wrinkles, when we make facial expressions. As we age, the fibroblasts lose their ability to make collagen and elastin. Other factors that affect our dermis is genetics, daily life decisions, and the environment. The bottom layer is called the subcutis or subcutaneous fat layer. As we age, our fatty layer begins to thin also leading to sagging.

Figure 15. Layers of the Skin (Can Stock Photo)

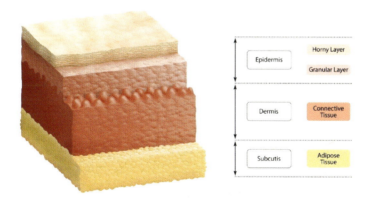

I always begin my physical exam by looking at the face, without the microscope, to determine if they have any signs that would contribute to DED. I know that skin conditions like rosacea and acne can damage the meibomian glands causing a poor fatty layer to the tear. I have also learned that skin damage due to smoking and sun exposure also negatively effects the tear glands.

Autoimmune diseases that have skin manifestations, such as scleroderma, psoriasis, dermatomyositis, epidermolysis bullosa, lupus, Sjogren's, and others, demonstrate to me that the disease or the medicines that they take for their disease could be the contributing to their dry eye. We know that Sjogren's diseases causes decrease production of water by the lacrimal gland, but the other autoimmune diseases cause dry eye as well, though not as publicized. The most common eye manifestation of Rhuematoid Arthritis is dry eye.

     After an adequate history and physical examination of the skin, I can begin to use the slit lamp (our examination microscope) to look at the lids. The most common sign I see with DED is telangiectasias that are associated with Rosacea. Many patients frequently deny that they have Rosacea because a dermatologist has told them that they do not have Rosacea, or when they think of the disease, they picture a patient with a red face, bulbous nose, and thinning skin. They do not have those signs, but Rosacea can have many degrees. The earliest sign is seeing telangiectasias along the thinnest skin of the body. These patients have these blood vessels throughout the face, but you can only detect them at the lids because the epidermis is thicker everywhere else, masking the telangiectasias. As these patients mature and their epidermis thins because of decrease collagen production and inflammatory breakdown then, the blood vessels will become more apparent. That is why some patients will say that they didn't have rosacea when they were younger, but now all of sudden, they contracted Rosacea. I warn these patients that as they become older their skin and dry eye will worsen without intervention. We began showing people their lid telangiectasias on a TV screen to demonstrate their Rosacea. Once identified, the patients are more proactive in caring for their skin by avoiding the sun, decrease in the use of acidic skin moisturizers, and eating foods that aggravate Rosacea like alcohol, inflammatory foods such as beef and dairy, starch, and sometimes caffeine. You should look for your personal trigger food. The skin and the telangiectasias secrete inflammatory mediators that breakdown the skin and the meibomian glands. If you can slow down the inflammation, then the patient's skin and meibomian glands will function better.

I counsel Rosacea patients to eat the Dry Eye Diet, like my other DED patients. They should also avoid warm compresses and lid scrubs because they agitate the telangiectasias and lead to more inflammation. Most commercially available moisturizers aggravate the skin because they were designed for normal skin. Skin products with a basic pH are less irritating to the skin in Rosacea patients. I find Kinerase and iScience (full disclosure - iScience is a Toyos Clinic product) skin products are well tolerated. In all patients, I recommend using skin products that will stimulate fibroblasts to produce collagen and elastin. In Rosacea patients, producing collagen will thicken the epidermis decreasing the vulnerability to the inflammatory mediators. Some products that clinical studies have shown to simulate fibroblasts are alpha hydroxys, antioxidants like Vitamin C, and retinoids. Some Rosacea patients find the retinoids irritating to the skin, so I suggest trying one before you buy it. One of the treatments for Rosacea is IPL not only because it closes telangiectasias, but it also stimulates fibroblasts.

Acne patients have a similar profile than Rosacea patients, and sometimes, the two diseases are together like in the disease Acne Rosacea. Acne appears at blocked skin pores. As we noted earlier, the top layer of dead skin cells slough off. Acne patients over produce the normal oil our skin utilizes to prevent drying called Sebum. The sebum causes the dead skin cells to stick together, blocking the pore. The gram positive bacteria that normally lives on the skin, propionibacterium acnes, can grow in the clogged pore causing redness, inflammation, and a pustule. The acne can be treated with benzoyl peroxide, salicylic acid, and blue LED. I have often seen Acne and MGD go hand in hand. A retinoid called Accutane[22] was prescribed for many years to control severe Acne. We have seen several dry eye patients with a history of Accutane use with dysfunctional glands. Accutane was linked to birth defects in women who utilized the drug during pregnancy and other side effects. Accutane was discontinued, but other generic forms are available. It was first thought that the dysfunctional meibomian glands in these Accutane patients were scarred down never to return to normal, but we have shown utilizing meibography that treatment with Intense Pulse Light can return these glands to normal.

Steven-Johnson is a rare reaction to medications that can affect the skin and mucous membranes. We have seen several patients with poor functioning meibomian glands, but we have been able to restore function with IPL. A similar problem has been reported in transplant patients that suffer from Graft Versus Host Disease GVHD. In this disease, the donor immune cells attack the recipient's body. We are studying IPL and other treatments for this disease.

The medications that patients take for autoimmune diseases can help or hurt DED. We covered some of the Biologics used in diseases like rheumatoid arthritis that are now being tried in DED. Some patients take oral steroids to help with their autoimmune problems. Unlike topical steroids that help the signs and symptoms of DED, oral steroids can exacerbate the DED[23]. We have found that same effect of topical NSAIDs versus oral NSAIDs. Table 1 and 2 reviews systemic and topical medications that may worsen DED symptoms.

Table 1. Systemic Medications.

SYSTEMIC MEDICATIONS		
ANTI-CHOLINERGIC	Antidepressants	SSRIs, TCAs, SNRIs, etc
	Antipyschotics/ Neuroleptics	
	Parkinson's Meds	1st and 2nd

NON ANTI-CHOLINERGIC	H-1 Antihistamines	generation Oral and Intranasal
	Decongestants	
	Overactive Bladder medications	
	H-2 Antihistamines/ Gastric Acting Drugs	
	Isoretinoin	Accutane
	Chemotherapeutics	
	Antihypertensives	Beta-blockers, Thiazides, ACE inhibitors, Angiotensin II receptor antagonist
	Anti-arrhythmics	
	Antithyroids	
	Opiod Analgesic	Morphine

Table 2. Topical Medications.

TOPICAL MEDICATIONS	
GLAUCOMA MEDICATION	Beta-blockers
	Adrenergic agonist
	Carbonic anhydrase inhibitors
	Cholinergic agents
	Prostaglandins
ANTIHISTAMINES	
ANTIVIRAL	
DECONGESTANTS	
MIOTICS	
MYDRIATICS AND CYCLOPLEGICS	
LOCAL ANESTHETICS	
NSAIDS	

Sun exposure can be the quickest way to aging skin because the Ultraviolet Light damages the elastin fibers in the skin. The skin without elastin will sag because it is missing the elasticity to spring back into place. The UV exposure can cause damage to the skin, including skin cancer. Blinking helps to push meibum from the glands. When the eyelids begin to sag, the force of the blink decreases, causing incomplete expression of the meibum. Some specialists train their patients to blink in a way that will create more force and express the glands. We can use medical grade skin products to stimulate more collagen, but sun damage is hard to reverse with medication. We have used fractional CO_2 lasers to resurface and tighten the skin of the face, including the eyelids. We have seen improved apposition of the lids and a more natural blink. Our clinic demonstrated improvement in TBUT with Mixto Laser Lift of the lids (treatment pioneered by Dr. Melissa Toyos). We are now performing laser facial rejuvenation and applying Platelet Rich Plasma to the skin for better healing and results.

As we age, we cannot stop the eyelids from drooping called dermatochalasis. When lasers fail to tighten the lids well enough, then a blepharoplasty, surgical excision of excess eyelid skin, is needed. You can perform the surgery with a scalpel or a laser. The surgery needs to performed accurately because if you remove too much of the eyelid skin, the patient cannot adequately close their eyes, causing exposure dry eye problems. Some surgeon's sacrifice function for a better cosmetic effect, but as we have seen for years, this could cause debilitating DED. When performing blepharoplasty, I would rather remove too little than too much skin. After blepharoplasty, if the patient would like a better cosmetic effect, we can utilize the laser to tighten the skin without causing exposure.

You can also have the lateral aspect of the lower eyelid droop, ectropion, because of dis-insertion of the lower lid retractors. You can have an exaggerated drooping of the lid that the layman will notice right away, but most patients have a mild case. The problem is that, even in the mild cases, it causes an incomplete blink. These patients have MGD of the lateral glands, causing a decreased fatty layer to their tear. In more severe cases, the patient will develop blepharitis and exposure keratitis (drying and scarring of the cornea).   Surgery to reinsert the lateral aspect of the lid can improve appearance but more importantly reestablish function of the lids to decrease the signs and symptoms of DED.

Smoking ages the skin prematurely because it increases free radicals in the body, destroying the normal maintenance of cellular processes. Even if you do not smoke, the production of free radicals is inevitable. We can decrease the amount of free radicals in our body with proper diet and supplements. Smoking overwhelms all of the healthy choices that you make in lifestyle. Smoking also narrows the normal blood vessels to the face, decreasing the oxygen supply. Smoking impedes the production of elastin and collagen.   One study showed smokers are twice as likely to have dry eyes. Smoke is an irritant, and studies have shown that it decreases the lipid layer of the tear film. Studies have shown that the number one way to stop patients from smoking is for a doctor to have a serious conversation with their patient about quitting. I advise you to follow the tips in this book, but it all starts with you not smoking.

The basics of helping your skin are simple, but I believe patients have a hard time adopting these solutions in their busy lives. We have shied away from over the counter skin products because if you are going to invest the time to take care of your skin, you should utilize medical grade products on the part of the skin that has the most exposure to the environment – the face. First, always cleanse, and occasionally exfoliate your skin. Every day, our skin comes in contact with a variety of environmental factors that can lead to inflammation that can expedite the aging process. Cleansers are the cornerstone of daily skin care. In many cases, a good cleanser can be all that is needed to polish a complexion, clear acne, or to even out a complexion. In every case, a good cleanser can improve both the moisture content and the effectiveness of any other product that you are using. Rosacea patients should pick a non-irritating cleanser with a basic pH.

AlphaBeta Cleanser, by iScience, contains natural alpha and beta hydroxyacids and salicylic acid to gently exfoliate oily and aging skins. These compounds naturally melt away the connections between old dead skin cells and literally allow you to rinse them away. Once the dead skin cells are removed, your skin will look smoother, softer and plumper, since it naturally retains more moisture once the old dead layer is no longer present to repel moisture.

How often should you cleanse? For dry skin, I recommend a gentle cleanser just once daily. Normal and oily skins usually benefit from a morning and evening cleanser. Water should be body temperature, not too cold or too hot to avoid irritation or aggravating rosacea tendencies.

You can occasionally exfoliate the skin with a treatment, like microdermabrasion, Intense Pulse Light, CO2, or Erbium Laser. Our clinic owns these technologies, but we do not utilize them often because the skin needs time to recover from these treatments. You need to let the fibroblasts time to generate collagen and elastin after a treatment to achieve the full effect. We have seen continued rejuvenation and improvement of the skin months after a Mixto Laser Lift.

Once your skin is clean, you can utilize a moisturizer to lock in water and other nutrients into the dermis.   As early as our 30's, we slow our production of the hyaluronic acid and some amino acids that not only plumps skin but acts as a sponge, pulling water in and holding it there. Without it, our skin looks thinner, less "plump" and dries out more easily. Hyaluronic acid can be replaced topically (it has been hard to get much in just by putting it on the skin). It is more easily put into the skin by injecting fillers, like Juvederm, to replace what has been lost.

Aging skin loses not only water content but also lipids and fat. Statistically, in our adult lives, we lose about 65% of the lipids in our skin that were present in our twenties. This is not only a loss of volume or fat in our faces but also a change in the character and texture of skin.

The change of life with hormonal fluctuations and loss of estrogen dramatically accelerates this process. Thinning skin tends to be most noticeable in the face, neck, chest, hands and forearms. We lose on average 6.4% of our total skin thickness with every passing decade. It only takes a few decades to really notice the changes.

We recommend MIXTOHydrate because it is the first moisturizer to pair acetyl-hexapeptide-37 and other peptides with hyaluronic acid to allow the hyaluronic acid to penetrate deeper into the skin than other products, where it can literally hydrate the skin from the inside out. One application of MIXTOHydrate will more than double your own skin hydration within 8 hours. Clinical studies show an unprecedented 131% increase in skin hydration 8 hours after using. With daily use, the same study showed that you can triple your skin's moisture content within 56 days. MIXTOHydrate also contains shea butter, squalene (natural lipid found in healthy young skin cells), and ceramides to lock in the moisture.

Another moisturizer with hyaluronic acid is iScience HydraPeptide Gel, a highly concentrated hyaluronic acid gel infused with vitamins B3, B5 and peptides. It is a unique formulation designed to not only enhance skin moisture but also to naturally improve the appearance of fine lines and dry skin. HydraPeptide gel also contains two different types of peptides that stimulate fibroblasts to make collagen and elastin to reduce fine lines and wrinkles from the inside out. It contains two separate compounds designed to inhibit skin enzymes generated by stress, pollution, and UV light that break down collagen and elastic fibers within the skin. Finally, the gel contains the powerful anti-oxidant – Green Tea.

Another moisturizer with different ingredients for sun and aged damaged skin is MixtoSilc by iScience. Made with a unique combination of naturally occurring skin moisturizers like ceramides, fatty acids and naturally occurring cholesterol, MIXTOSilc replaces essential oils in the skin lost from age, harsh products, lack of proper hydration and the dry, cold air of winter. Enhanced with olive derived squalene, MIXTOSilc restores the ideal moisture balance to dry, inflamed, and aging skin without fragrance or preservatives to make it safe for even the most sensitive of skins.

    After the moisturizer, you need to sun protect your skin. I recommend sun blocks that have not one but two physical sun blockers to block the UVA rays associated with aging and the UVB rays that burn the skin.   The iScience products contain these products for comprehensive sun protection, but they also contain a transparent melanin (the same thing that is naturally found in your skin to protect you against the sun) so that UV rays are absorbed on top of your skin before they get to your skin at all. It is the only product made that contains all of these safeguards and none of the dangerous chemicals found in some sunscreens that can disrupt natural hormone balances.

    What we eat can also sun protect and maintain healthy skin. Along with my recommended DED diet, you can include these foods. A study published in the European Journal of Cancer Prevention demonstrated an 11% lower prevalence of non-melanoma skin cancer in women who drank coffee everyday as those who did not drink coffee. When you're drinking your coffee, you can have some filtered water, a medium sized kiwi, and pumpkin seeds. The kiwi will give you 120% of your daily requirement of Vitamin C. Vitamin C stimulates the fibroblasts to produce collagen. Pumpkin seeds are a great source of Zinc, an important mineral in many cells of our body including the skin and eyes. Many individuals are deficient in Zinc, due to the mineral depleted soils. Pumpkin seeds can also stabilize hormones in post-menopausal women since they are a rich source of phytoestrogens. Studies have shown phytoestrogen supplementation in women can improve the signs and symptoms of DED[25].

    A study in the journal, Cornea[26] showed no statistical difference in the blood levels of B12 in DED patients versus patient without DED, but B12 is necessary in normal functioning of all cells. Patients with B12 deficiency will notice skin changes first, like hyper or hypopigmentation spots. Your body cannot produce B12 on its own, necessitating dietary supplementation. B12 is not produced in plants, so vegans have a difficult time obtaining enough B12. Mackerel is one of the best sources of vitamin B12, containing 16 mcg, or 270% of what your body needs in a day. Other sources that fit into the DED diet are salmon and sardines.

"Strength does not come from physical capacity. It comes from an indomitable will."

    Gandhi (1869-1948)

Chapter 9: Aging

I have always realized the importance of staying in shape to my overall wellness. My mind tells me that I can still accomplish physically all the activities that I could when I was 20, but heading into my 50's, I know that I cannot still dunk a basketball with little effort, preparation, and conditioning. We can accept that other parts of our body's age and function less effectively, but when it comes to our eyes, it is a different story. We want our glands that secrete the tear film to work the same throughout our lifespan. We demonstrated that our skin produces less collagen as we age. I have seen in our clinic that with increasing age, our meibomian and lacrimal glands do not produce the same tear film. Most of my patients tell me that they didn't always have dry eye, but as they aged, the symptoms became worse. Factors that contribute to the problem are years of inflammation, skin changes, and poor diet and conditioning. In women, hormonal changes contribute to the problem but not to the point that oral or topical hormones have helped.

A substantial amount of money is being spent studying the aging process and how to slow down the ill effects. For DED, we can look at the aging process of our glands that produce the tear film at the cellular and genetic level. We know at the cellular level, we can apply treatments to perk up the slowing cellular metabolism. We know that Intense Pulse Light and Light Emitting Diodes can stimulate the mitochondria of cells to work more efficiently. The light treatments that I have invented cause the meibomian and lacrimal glands to produce better secretions. The glands and lids of patients that have IPL for years look better compared to similar patients their own age that have not had IPL treatments. We know that certain dietary supplements, like antioxidants, can stimulate cellular function. Antioxidants and retinoids can stimulate the fibroblasts to produce elastin and collagen. I believe if you follow the insights given in the book, your cellular function will be improved.

What happens to us genetically as we age? Our chromosomes go through cell division throughout our lives. Telomeres are short DNA segments that are not responsible for cellular code but are there as buffers, to protect the necessary DNA for replication. The telomeres shorten with each cell division. Eventually, the telomeres are so short they can no longer protect the DNA during division, causing malfunction and death. Telomere length has been shown to be a good predictive indicator for life expectancy. Ground breaking research is going on to elongate these telomeres to the length seen in youth. One company, Bioviva, has been applying gene therapy to humans in the hopes of increasing telomere length. I am not advocating gene therapy at this point, but can we do something now?

A University of California of San Francisco study showed that the higher the fish derived Omega-3 fatty acids in the blood of coronary artery disease patients, the longer the telomeres. Another reason to increase the salmon intake. A twin study published in the Archives of Internal Medicine demonstrated that the twin that exercised had longer telomeres than the sedentary ones. I recommend that my patients incorporate a walking program because it satisfies the exercise requirement and decreases stress. The Okinawans, who are famous for long life, don't use stairmasters or weights. They just walk everywhere. The Chinese herb, astragalus, contains astragalosides and cycloastragenols, enzymes that stimulate telomerase enzyme. The telomerase helps regeneration of the telomere and can be found in two patented forms – TAT2 and TA-65. Vitamin D from the sun or as a supplement can slow the rate of shortening of the telomeres. The final anti-aging tip may be the most controversial.

Many studies have shown that drinking alcohol in moderation may lead to a longer life. Alcohol has been shown to reduce the risk of atherosclerosis and reduction in coronary artery disease. Most health experts recommend a small glass of red wine a few times a week as the alcohol of choice because it contains resveratrol. A Malbec has the most resveratrol because the grape has the thickest skin. Resveratrol was shown to increase the life of yeast by 60 percent[24]. Harvard Medical School showed that mice given resveratrol lived longer than their cohorts. Before you say that I blessed your wine habit, you can get resveratrol by eating red grapes.

A more bioavailable resveratrol-like supplement is pterostilbene. Some studies have shown that in mice, pterostilbene is more potent in improving brain function and preventing cancer and heart disease. Four times more pterostilbene is found in the bloodstream than resveratrol. Dr. Leonard Guarente at the MIT Glenn Lab for the Science of Aging has developed a supplement that has combined pterostilbene with Nicotinamide Riboside, a precursor to nicotinamide adenine dinucleotide, NAD. NAD has been shown in animal models to aide our cellular mitochondria produce energy. As we age, our mitochondria slow down, and our NAD levels decline. Harvard's David Sinclair lab reported that injecting elderly mice with a NAD booster restored the mitochondria of their muscle. NAD and resveratrol improve the function of enzymes that helped mice counter the bad effects of a high fat diet called sirtuins. The more NAD, the more mitochondria are formed and the better they run. More research is being completed on these supplements, but the work is encouraging.

I have DED patients, female and male, that utilize anti-aging human growth hormone and testosterone replacement. I have seen a difference in their physical appearance including in their skin, but I have not seen a positive effect on their DED. We are in the early stages of seeing how human growth hormone will fit into the anti-aging armamentarium and if it can have any effect on dry eye. I believe we have too many other anti-aging options at this point to jump in blindly into hormone replacement. One hormone that has been studied many times but still rears its head periodically is testosterone cream for DED. I had a front row seat to the testosterone cream experiments for dry eye because it was advocated and studied by Dr. Connor, previously at the Southern College of Optometry in Memphis. Earlier studies by Dr. Sullivan and others showed that androgens could play a role in the function of the Meibomian and Lacrimal glands. Dr. Connor then tried various concentrations of transdermal testosterone cream to improve DED without significant efficacy. Since one of my clinics is in Memphis, many of my patients took part in these studies. His studies did not show significant improvement. Many female patients complained of hair growth in unwanted parts of their body. I think the initial studies showing a link to hormones and gland function were interesting but extrapolating this research to a treatment never materialized. Even with this, I see this treatment reappear over and over. If I see this reappear again in 2020 without any studies to back it up, I will be disappointed but not surprised.

"We made buttons on the screen look so good you'll want to lick them."

      Steve Jobs (1955-2011)

Chapter 10: Environment

Take a break from your phone for one second

    In the age of handheld electronics, computers, screen entertainment, and visually focused employment, it would seem that everyone is at risk of dry eye. I often tell my patients with any visually engrossing task, your blink rate will be reduced. We conducted a study where we looked at normal patients under the age of 30 who did not have DED and measured their TBUT. We found that some of these patients could achieve TBUT's up to 30 seconds. The normal blink is about every 10 seconds.

    When a person is completing a visual task, whether it is reading a book or tablet, the blink rate is less frequent. As we stated, we found young healthy patients that could keep a normal tear on their eye for 30 seconds, so it easy to see where extending the time between blinks will not be as much of a problem. Several problems are arising because we have a growing number of people with MGD, and they cannot keep a normal tear on their eye as long. When they are completing these visual tasks, they are now feeling their DED because they are overwhelming their system. A patient with borderline normal TBUT of 10 seconds, when asked to complete visual tasks that require them to keep their eyes open longer, now find themselves with symptoms of dry eye. We often have patients who will visit the clinic and say that they never had problems with dry eye until they started this new job. When we question these patients, they admit that their new job requires staring at a computer all day, or if they work in a manufacturing plant, they are performing a visual task that requires concentration, whereas before their job didn't require the amount of visual concentration. We had a professional baseball player with DED, and his hitting was suffering because his TBUT was less than 5 seconds so he compensated for the short TBUT by blinking more. Of course, his frequent blinking caused him to misjudge pitches decreasing his hitting productivity; we improved his hitting by improving his MGD.

We conducted a study where we utilized an artificial tear to see if we could help normal baseball players visual performance. We found even in normal patients without DED who perform jobs that require visual concentration and longer blink times that lubricating their eyes before work helped their visual performance.

If you have MGD and DED, you need to realize that you cannot extend your blink rate easily, and you have to make adjustments. I perform many of my surgeries under the microscope, and when you are working in the eye, you really can't afford to blink many times. I use an artificial tear before have a long day of surgery so that my visual performance won't suffer later in the day. I also force myself to allow my eyes a break between surgeries. For me, it as simple as closing my eyes for a few minutes a couple of times a day. In Japan, desk workers are required to take periodic breaks where they close and rest their eyes.

As we stated before, the blink is necessary to help release the meibum from the meibomian gland. Some patients suffer from an incomplete blink; instead of bringing the lids together to express the glands, they barely close their eyes. Now, I have seen this after improper lid surgery where too much skin is removed, prohibiting the patient to close their eyes fully, but I have also seen it in patients who have no anatomical and functional problem. Some of these patients can be taught to blink properly. I want to make sure that you understand that this is rare condition. Some doctors waste time having all their patients go through blink training.

I believe the best philosophy is to instruct patients on the importance of the blink and taking time from all the digital gadgets to rest the eyes and to explain to patients that artificial tears will never cure your dry eye problem. You can use them to help you during those times when you need support during work and studying, and you can't necessarily take a break.

Allergy

Environmental allergies will exacerbate the signs and symptoms of DED. Some of the same inflammatory mediators found in the tear of patients with DED are also found in patients with allergic conjunctivitis. One reason why we cannot find a definite test for DED looking at the mediators in the tear film is the presence of these mediators in allergy. If a patient tests for an elevated MMP-9, is it because the patient has an allergy or MGD?

In a normal exam, we ask if the patient has been diagnosed with an environmental allergy. We determine if the allergy is seasonal or perennial. Are they taking medications or eye drops for their allergies? Many of the oral antihistamines, like Allegra and Claritin, can dry the eyes (see the list of medications that dry the eyes). Many of the antihistamine eye drops dry the eyes as well.

During the exam, we determine if they have DED and allergic conjunctivitis. If they have both, we attack this problem very differently than most specialists. I will stop all drops that are proven to make dry eye worse. I stop all drops that have a preservative. I want to see what their eyes look like without these compounding factors. If they can survive without oral medications that dry them out, then I will stop them. I have the patient practice avoidance of all possible allergens. For example, if they are allergic to their dog, then they shouldn't let the dog sleep in the bed or even hang out in the bedroom. Most patients cannot avoid many of their surroundings, but what they can do is keep from bringing their surroundings with them to bed. In a normal day, allergens will accumulate in the hair, and when the patient goes to sleep their face and eyes will be rolling in them, causing inflammation all night long without a chance for relief. I suggest showering at night, including washing the hair. For added protection of the eyes, they can use a strip of Glad Press and Seal placed tight on closed eyelids. (This is also a great trick for patients who do not have complete closure of the eyelids when they sleep.) The only drop that they can use is a preservative free artificial tear when necessary. Then, we begin treating their DED.

On a return visit, we check to see the true extend of their eye allergies. We schedule the appointment in the morning to see if our tricks are at least decreasing the allergy overnight. Sometimes, we find that our interventions are enough to control the eye allergy. If it is not enough, then we prescribe Bepreve drops, an antihistamine drop that we noticed clinically did not dry the eyes, twice a day. We also noticed that Bepreve cleared the sinuses of some patients with topical application.

The advantage of treating DED with technologies like IPL is that the patients stop drops that have preservatives. Then, if for some reason, you need to use a drop like Bepreve that has BAK, which can cause allergies, you have made the environment less toxic. If the patient does have a BAK allergy, you will know with our protocol because they have stopped all other drops except preservative free artificial tears.

We have not found allergy shots helpful in our DED and allergy patients.

"The philosophies of one age have become the absurdities of the next, and the foolishness of yesterday has become the wisdom of tomorrow."

 Sir William Osler (1849-1919)

Chapter 11: Treatments that didn't make the cut

  In one of the Star Trek movies with the original cast, the doctor character, Bones, time travels back to the past. He walks in a hospital and walks by a patient in serious pain on a stretcher. His curiosity takes over, and he looks at the chart. The patient is scheduled to have surgery of a tumor on the brain. Bones reads the chart and yells something to the effect of how could these butchers do this barbaric surgery to this poor woman. He pulls out his futuristic handheld healing device and waves it around the patient's head, and instantly, the patient is cured and walking off the gurney. I wonder what the doctors will say about some of the treatments that have been offered today. I developed this section because I know that financial resources are limited and do not want patients to waste money on treatments that are being utilized today and, in my experience, have not been worth the money.

  Some doctors have been advocating using an electric toothbrush device to clean the lids. When a patient has blepharitis, she will have a build-up of bacteria and demodex on the lid margin. These microorganisms produce lipases that destroy the lipid layer of the tear film as well as cause inflammation that impair the meibomian glands. What comes first the blepharitis or the DED? They are linked together at the hip. Cleaning the lids at the doctor's office will not solve the underlying problem because the bacteria repopulate. If you are combining the cleaning with another treatment, you will get some benefit. I have to admit that I tried the treatment. The agitation caused inflammation of the lids. I tell patients not to perform lid scrubs because the agitation of the vigorous scrubbing of the lids causes the vessels of the area to dilate and bring inflammatory mediators to the area, providing a counterproductive effect.

A procedure that made the rounds about ten years ago but has not completely died out is meibomian gland probing. Some doctors thought that the problem with the meibomian glands is that they are scarred down, and that is the reason no meibum would be released when pushed on. When I started showing my videos of post-IPL expression showing toothpaste-like secretions sprouting from once silent glands, doctors realized that the glands were not dormant but packed with thick abnormal meibum, blocking the glands. We showed that glands that had dropped out because of lack of secretion could be revived with IPL. Scarred down glands were rare, so probing did not serve a purpose but could also cause damage, if not done carefully. I can only imagine what Bones would say if he walked in on this procedure.

I am going to put the plethora of DED diagnostics in this category. I am not going to single out any of them. We know that DED is a multifactorial disease, and as my wife states, "we do not have the pregnancy test of DED", where one simple test tells you yes or no definitively. Returning to the story where a "DED specialist" had a DED patient go through a battery of expensive tests. Some tests were positive, others negative, and some unequivocal. In the end, after all these tests, the doctor treated based on signs and symtoms. We cannot impede progress, but we should not waste precious health care dollars on tests that will not change our clinical judgment. These tests should still be in the experimental phase until it can be a simple yes or no answer. Then, if the answer is no, it has to mean that it changes our treatment paradigm. There was a saying when I went to medical school – "treat the patient, not the test".

"Somewhere, something incredible is waiting to be known."

Carl Sagan (1934-1996)

Chapter 12: The Future in Dry Eye

When patients ask what is the ultimate future for the treatment of dry eye disease, I often tell them the future of all disease treatment will be in gene manipulation. Famous outspoken futurist, Ray Kurzweil, PhD, often lectures on exponential advancements in all specialties that involve information technology. For example, think about the computing power of our desktop computer 10 years ago as compared to the computing power of our handheld phone today. The same exponential growth is happening in genomics. The Human Genome Project started in 1990, and by 1997, only 1 percent of the mapping of our DNA had been accomplished. Dr. Kurzweil points out that in exponential progression if you double 1 percent seven more times, you would get 100 percent in a few years, and that is exactly what happened. The Human Genome Project was completed in 2003 at a cost of a billion dollars. Now, I can have my patient's DNA mapped by a company, such as 23 and Me, for less than 300 dollars.

Once the genes are mapped, we can pinpoint which sequences are responsible for specific human functions. You can now find out if you are predisposed to certain diseases. You have seen genetic testing play out in women being tested for the BRCA1 breast cancer gene to determine their risk. Some high risk women have had mastectomies performed based on their genetic information. Couples can use genetic testing to see if they have a high risk of passing on a disease to a child. For example, you can find out if you and your spouse are a carrier for cystic fibrosis. If two carriers were to have a child, their risk of having a child with cystic fibrosis is increased dramatically over the general population.

The genetic information from mapping can help us unlock some of the genetic causes of dry eye.

DED is common with specific diseases, like Sjogren's Syndrome and Rosacea. Sjogren's syndrome is an autoimmune disorder where the immune system attacks one's own body. Patients with the disease have their lacrimal and salivary glands attacked by antibodies and immune cells. A small percentage of DED patients have this disorder, affecting the water production in tears. Several genes have been identified like IRF5, BLK, and TNFAIP3 to name a few. Researchers at Stanford University have identified a genetic basis for Rosacea. Dr. Anne Lynn Chang, MD et al. published a paper that demonstrated a link between Rosacea and genetic variants of the HLA-DRA and BTNL2 genes[18]. We explained how Rosacea patients are more prone to MGD Dry Eye Disease earlier.

Once you know the gene that is responsible for a particular disease, research can be completed to decrease the expression of the bad gene or, in time, correct the gene. For example, Phenylketonuria (PKU) is an autosomal recessive disorder caused by the deficiency of phenylalanine hydroxylase (PAH). These patients cannot metabolize an amino acid in protein found in food. Researchers discovered mutations in the PAH gene in these patients. People without PKU use the phenylalanine in food and break down the excess with PAH. Patients with PKU cannot break phenylalanine down, causing toxic levels in the brain and impairing development. PKU patients can live normal lives with strict restriction of phenylalanine in their diet and supplementing with a medical formula containing amino acids. Now, think for a second how manageable DED would be if we found the gene responsible for dry eye, and we determined it can be controlled similar to PKU with a change of diet or environment. For example, I have had plenty of dry eye patients tell me that their dry eye improved with some modifications to their diet. We know that MGD DED patients with Rosacea respond to diets that have fewer foods that are pro-inflammatory. Also, we know that certain environmental factors may trigger a genetic manifestation of dry eye. It could be attributed to allergy, but what if it was something more? For example, patients on birth control pills have a higher risk of breast cancer than patients who have never used birth control; the hormones could activate the breast cancer gene.

We are living in the time that bad genes can and will be fixed. In the disease Severe Combined Immune Deficiency (Adenosine Deaminase Deficiency) ADA-SCID, also known as bubble boy disease, children have a defect in their immune system that decreases their ability to fight off simple infections. The most common form of SCID patients will have a defect in the SCIDX1 gene. There is a documented cure utilizing gene manipulation to cure the disease. A therapeutic gene called ADA was introduced into the bone marrow cells of patients in the lab. Then, the genetically corrected cells were injected back into the patients, successfully curing them of their disease. Once we have complete mapping of DED, ways to correct these genes will be discovered.

As DED affects more and more of our population, we will see more money invested in true treatments and cures. I have seen the exponential growth in dollars supporting DED research. I can't remember over the last 10 years when we have not had an FDA or a Biotech company sponsored DED study. My feeling is that we went from 0 to 60 in a short time. I am hopeful that we will continue to progress in the next four years, so that we will say that patients, doctors, and researchers came together to control Dry Eye Disease by the year 2020.

Bibliography

1. Lemp, Michael A., MD, and Gary N. Foulks, MD. "The Definition & Classification of Dry Eye Disease: Guidelines from the 2007 International Dry Eye Workshop." *Tear Film and Ocular Surface Society* (2008): n. pag. Apr. 2008. Web.
2. "SPIE." *The International Society for Optics and Photonics*. SPIE, 2016. Web. 10 Apr. 2016.
3. "The Optical Society." *OSA*. The Optical Society, 2016. Web. 10 Apr. 2016.
4. Roy, Steve, ed. *NASA Light Technology Successfully Reduces Cancer Patients Painful Side Effects from Radiation and Chemotherapy*. Publication. NASA, 3 Mar. 2011. Web.
5. Wise, Ryan J., Rachel K. Sobel, and Richard C. Allen. "Meibography: A Review of Techniques and Technologies." *Saudi Journal of Ophthalmology* 26.4 (2012): 349-56.
6. Terada, O. "Ocular Surface Temperature of Meibomian Gland Dysfunction Patients and the Melting Point of Meibomian Gland Secretions." *Nippon Ganka Gakkai Zasshi* 108.11 (2004): 690-93. Print.
7. Stibich, Mark, Julie Stachowiak, Benjamin Tanner, Matthew Berkheiser, Linette Moore, Issam Raad, and Roy F. Chemaly. "Evaluation of a Pulsed-Xenon Ultraviolet Room Disinfection Device for Impact on Hospital Operations and Microbial Reduction." *Infect Control Hosp Epidemiol Infection Control & Hospital Epidemiology* 32.03 (2011): 286-88.
8. Maisch, Tim, Franz Spannberger, Johannes Regensburger, Ariane Felgenträger, and Wolfgang Bäumler. "Fast and Effective: Intense Pulse Light Photodynamic Inactivation of Bacteria." *Journal of Industrial Microbiology & Biotechnology J Ind Microbiol Biotechnol* 39.7 (2012): 1013-021
9. Fodor, Lucian, Yehuda Ullmann, and Monica Elman. *Aesthetic Applications of Intense Pulsed Light*. London: Springer, 2011. Print.

10. Fox, Robert I., Raymond Chan, Joseph B. Michelson, Jonathan B. Belmont, and Paul E. Michelson. "Beneficial Effect of Artificial Tears Made with Autologous Serum in Patients with Keratoconjunctivitis Sicca." *Arthritis & Rheumatism* 27.4 (1984): 459-61. Web.
11. Tsubota, K., E. Goto, H. Fujita, M. Ono, H. Inoue, I. Saito, and S. Shimmura. "Treatment of Dry Eye by Autologous Serum Application in Sjogren's Syndrome." *British Journal of Ophthalmology* 83.4 (1999): 390-95. Web.
12. Paiva, Cintia S. De, Zhuo Chen, Douglas D. Koch, M. Bowes Hamill, Francis K. Manuel, Sohela S. Hassan, Kirk R. Wilhelmus, and Stephen C. Pflugfelder. "The Incidence and Risk Factors for Developing Dry Eye After Myopic LASIK." *American Journal of Ophthalmology* 141.3 (2006): 438-45. Web.
13. "TruPRP." *Magellan*. Arteriocyte Medical Systems, Inc, 2016. Web.
14. Viola, Publio, and Marzia Viola. "Virgin Olive Oil as a Fundamental Nutritional Component and Skin Protector." *Clinics in Dermatology* 27.2 (2009): 159-65. Web.
15. Lobo, V., A. Patil, A. Phatak, and N. Chandra. "Free Radicals, Antioxidants and Functional Foods: Impact on Human Health." *Pharmacognosy Reviews Phcog Rev* 4.8 (2010): 118. Web.
16. Arita, Reiko, Yasuo Yanagi, Norihiko Honda, Shuji Maeda, Koshi Maeda, Aya Kuchiba, Takuhiro Yamaguchi, Yoshitsugu Yanagihara, Hiroshi Suzuki, and Shiro Amano. "Caffeine Increases Tear Volume Depending on Polymorphisms within the Adenosine A2a Receptor Gene and Cytochrome P450 1A2." *Ophthalmology* 119.5 (2012): 972-78. Web.
17. "Anakinra." *Kineret* (2003): n. pag. *FDA*. Web.
18. Chang, Anne Lynn S., Inbar Raber, Jin Xu, Rui Li, Robert Spitale, Julia Chen, Amy K. Kiefer, Chao Tian, Nicholas K. Eriksson, David A. Hinds, and Joyce Y. Tung. "Assessment of

the Genetic Basis of Rosacea by Genome-Wide Association Study." *Journal of Investigative Dermatology* 135.6 (2015): 1548-555. Web
19. Neubronner, J., et al., "Enhanced increase of omega-3 index in response to long-term n-3 fatty acid supplementation from triacylglycerides versus ethyl esters." *Eur J Clin Nutr*, 2011. 65(2): 247-54.
20. Tokudome, S., et al., "Japanese versus Mediterranean Diets and Cancer." *Asian Pac J Cancer Prev*, 2000. 1(1): 61-66. *PubMed*. Web. 2016.
21. Albietz, Julie M., and Lee M. Lenton. "Effect of Antibacterial Honey on the Ocular Flora in Tear Deficiency and Meibomian Gland Disease." *Cornea* 25.9 (2006): 1012-019. Web.
22. Wong, John, Wanwen Lan, Li Ming Ong, and Louis Tong. "Non-hormonal Systemic Medications and Dry Eye." *The Ocular Surface* 9.4 (2011): 212-26. Web.
23. Fraunfelder, Frederick T., James J. Sciubba, and William D. Mathers. "The Role of Medications in Causing Dry Eye." *Journal of Ophthalmology* 2012 (2012): 1-8. Web.
24. Howitz, Konrad T., Kevin J. Bitterman, Haim Y. Cohen, Dudley W. Lamming, Siva Lavu, Jason G. Wood, Robert E. Zipkin, Phuong Chung, Anne Kisielewski, Li-Li Zhang, Brandy Scherer, and David A. Sinclair. "Small Molecule Activators of Sirtuins Extend Saccharomyces Cerevisiae Lifespan." *Nature* 425.6954 (2003): 191-96. Web.
25. Scuderi, Gianluca, Maria Teresa Contestabile, Caterina Gagliano, Daniela Iacovello, Luca Scuderi, and Teresio Avitabile. "Effects of Phytoestrogen Supplementation in Postmenopausal Women with Dry Eye Syndrome: A Randomized Clinical Trial." *Canadian Journal of Ophthalmology / Journal Canadien D'Ophtalmologie* 47.6 (2012): 489-92. Web.

26. Sekeryapan, Berrak, Veysi Oner, Aynur Kirbas, Kemal Turkyilmaz, and Mustafa Durmus. "Plasma Homocysteine Levels in Dry Eye Patients." *Cornea* 32.5 (2013): n. pag. Web.
27. "Health Starts with Science." *Elysium Health*. N.p., n.d. Web. 28 Apr. 2016
28. Moscovici, Bernardo K., Ricardo Holzchuh, Brenda B. Chiacchio, Ruth M. Santo, Jun Shimazaki, and Richard Y. Hida. "Clinical Treatment of Dry Eye Using 0.03% Tacrolimus Eye Drops." *Cornea* 31.8 (2012): 945-49. Web.
29. Pucci, Neri, Roberto Caputo, Laura Di Grande, Cinzia De Libero, Francesca Mori, Simona Barni, Lorena Di Simone, Annamaria Calvani, Franca Rusconi, and Elio Novembre. "Tacrolimus vs. Cyclosporine Eyedrops in Severe Cyclosporine-resistant Vernal Keratoconjunctivitis: A Randomized, Comparative, Double-blind, Crossover Study." *Pediatr Allergy Immunol Pediatric Allergy and Immunology* 26.3 (2015): 256-61. Web.
30. Younger, Jarred, Luke Parkitny, and David Mclain. "The Use of Low-dose Naltrexone (LDN) as a Novel Anti-inflammatory Treatment for Chronic Pain." *Clin Rheumatol Clinical Rheumatology* 33.4 (2014): 451-59. Web.

Testimonials from patients

"I am in Napa. I had to get up yesterday at 3:30am, fly to Frisco, and then drive to Napa. My dry eyes feel great thanks to Rolando Toyos and his dry eye treatment. You have definitely improved my quality of life."

"I have been to multiple other clinics with no relief for my severe dry eyes. However, since receiving treatment by Dr. Toyos I have notice improvements in my dry eyes. I would highly recommend Dr. Toyos to anyone with skin or eye care needs!"

"Thank you for helping my dry eye disease. I have reason to live now without pain all the time"

About the Author

Rolando Toyos, M.D. is the Medical Director and Founder of Toyos Clinic. He received his Bachelors and Masters degrees from The University of California, Berkeley and Stanford University. He received his medical degree at the University of Illinois, graduating with James Scholar Academic Honors and received a community service award for helping Chicago City Public Schools develop a pre-med program for students interested in medicine. He completed his internship in Internal Medicine at Illinois Masonic Hospital in Chicago. He completed his Ophthalmology residency at Northwestern University and Chicago Children's Hospital. He has authored several papers and books, including *The Insider's Guide to Medical School Admissions* and *The Life and Times of a Sports Ophthalmologist*. He has lectured and trained Ophthalmologists about Dry Eye Disease around the world. He has presented his research internationally at ISOPT, APAO, ASCRS, ESCRS and AAO to name a few. Dr. Toyos has received several awards, including the ASCRS award and the Humanitarian Award from the Jazz Foundation of America. For fun, Dr. Toyos loves spending time with his wife, Dr. Melissa Toyos, an award winning Ophthalmologist, and their three girls.

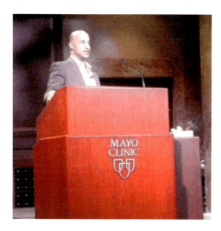
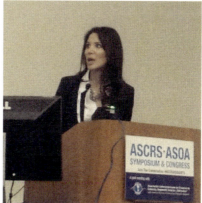

Made in the USA
Columbia, SC
09 January 2020

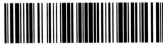